**C.M.B Questions**
**and How to Answer T**

4-1-82.

# C.M.B. QUESTIONS
## and How to Answer Them

## Vera da Cruz, SRN, SCM, MTD

*formerly Principal Tutor Queen Charlotte's Maternity Hospital
and Examiner to the Central Midwives Board*

FABER AND FABER

London · Boston

First published in 1956
by Faber and Faber Limited
3 Queen Square London WC1
Second edition 1959
Third edition 1961
Fourth edition 1969
Reprinted 1972
Fifth edition 1977
Reprinted 1979 and 1981
Printed in Great Britain by
Whitstable Litho Ltd, Whitstable
All rights reserved

ISBN 0 571 04919 2

# Preface to the Fifth Edition

Midwifery practice and, with it, teaching and examinations change, often imperceptibly and usually more quickly than we realise. Knowledge increases, fresh ideas are evolved, technological data come to be accepted as part of day-to-day routine and the very language of our profession alters.

Midwifery training approaches the end of a much more radical change. Single period training is the rule, first period training is over and second period training is being phased out more gradually. Examination papers of the sixties are often so outdated that, in a small book dealing solely with this subject, extensive revision is obviously necessary.

The Central Midwives Board Examination at present consists of a three-hour Midwifery and Paediatrics paper and a two-hour Community Health paper, followed three weeks later by a twenty-minute oral examination. The examinations of the Central Midwives Board for Scotland and the Northern Ireland Council for Nurses and Midwives are similar, but not identical; in the former, two two-hour papers are followed by a thirty-minute clinical and oral examination; the latter comprises a three-hour paper and an oral, clinical and practical examination. The clinical part of the examination has, over the years, become increasingly difficult to administer. Its value, though not invalidated, is open to question and it may, in the future, be discontinued.

I would like to acknowledge most gratefully the continued courtesy of the Central Midwives Board, whose examination papers have furnished material for the major part of this edition.

I am greatly appreciative, too, to be able again to include a number of questions from the papers set by comparable examining bodies and my grateful thanks are due to the Central Midwives Board for Scotland and the Northern Ireland Council for Nurses and Midwives for their ready co-operation.

Throughout this revision I have been deeply grateful to Miss P. J. Cunningham, BA, SRN, SCM, HVCert, of Faber and Faber Ltd, for much valued advice and assistance.

Richmond, Surrey February 1976                    Vera da Cruz

# Contents

# Illustrations

# The Central Midwives Board's Examinations

# The Central Midwives Board's Examinations

## THE CENTRAL MIDWIVES BOARD'S AND COMPARABLE EXAMINATIONS

Single Period midwifery training was introduced experimentally in 1968, the first Integrated Examination being held in 1969. The experimental period proved successful, the training quickly became popular and, in recent years, it has been introduced much more extensively, while First and Second Period training are gradually being phased out.

Both the Central Midwives Board for Scotland and the Northern Ireland Council for Nurses and Midwives were able to effect an immediate change, partly because far fewer training schools were involved and partly because they were concerned with one training only: the twelve months' training for State Registered Nurses and Registered General Nurses.

Though not identical, the three examinations have many similar features.

The English examination consists of two written papers, a three-hour Midwifery and Paediatrics paper and a two-hour Community Health paper, followed three weeks later by a twenty-minute oral examination. The papers are marked by a consultant obstetrician and a midwife teacher who also conduct the oral examination.

The candidate brings to the oral examination three case studies which she has herself compiled, of patients whom she has delivered, and subsequently attended and followed up until the 28th postnatal day. Each case study is required to contain a summary of not more than 200 words, illustrating how medical, social and environmental factors may have influenced the care given to mother and baby. One or more of these case studies is discussed during the oral examination.

The Scottish examination is on similar lines, having two two-hour papers, one on Midwifery and the other on Paediatrics and Community Health, with, at present, a clinical/oral examination of 30 minutes duration.

The Northern Ireland pattern of examination differs only in a few respects, the three-hour paper being followed by a clinical, oral and practical session.

The question papers from three recent examinations are set out below.

### Central Midwives Board

INTEGRATED EXAMINATION – MIDWIFERY AND PAEDIATRICS

*17th September 1975 from 2.00 p.m. to 5.00 p.m.*

*PART I – One Hour – Candidates should answer both questions*

1. Describe the anatomy of the uterus.
   What changes does the uterus undergo in pregnancy and labour?
2. What are the funtions of the placenta?
   How may placental function be monitored in pregnancy?

*PART II – Two hours – Write about 50 words on each of the following:*

3. (a) Vomiting in pregnancy.
   (b) Vaginal discharge in pregnancy.
   (c) High head at term in a primigravida.
   (d) Abdominal X-rays in pregnancy.
4. (a) Ketosis in labour.
   (b) Occipito-posterior positions in labour.
   (c) Analgesic drugs in labour.
   (d) Meconium staining in the amniotic fluid.
5. (a) Hypernatraemia in the neonate.
   (b) Ophthalmia neonatorum.
   (c) Cerebral irritation in the newborn.
   (d) The use of the incubator.

6. (a) Urinary complications in the puerperium.
   (b) Significance of lochia.
   (c) Breast feeding.
   (d) Secondary postpartum haemorrhage.

*CANDIDATES SHOULD NOTE THAT ANSWERS SHOULD BE CON-
CISE AND THAT EXTRA MARKS WILL <u>NOT</u> BE GIVEN FOR ANSWERS
OF MORE THAN 50 WORDS IN PART II OF THE PAPER.

### Central Midwives Board

INTEGRATED EXAMINATION – COMMUNITY HEALTH

*17th September 1975 from 10.00 a.m. to 12.00 noon*

*PART I – One Hour – Candidates should answer any two of these
questions*

1. Discuss the problems of one-parent families.
   What help is available to them?
2. Why is community care included in the training of a midwife?
   Discuss the value of this experience.
3. Discuss the regulations concerning child adoption.

*PART II – One Hour – Write about 50 words on each of the
following*

1. Immunisation programme for children up to five years of age.
2. The role of the husband in the puerperium.
3. Attendance allowance.
4. Environmental Health Inspector.
5. Battered baby syndrome.
6. Perinatal mortality.
7. Citizens Advice Bureau.
8. Area Health Authorities.

*CANDIDATES SHOULD NOTE THAT ANSWERS SHOULD BE CON-
CISE AND THAT EXTRA MARKS WILL <u>NOT</u> BE GIVEN FOR ANSWERS
OF MORE THAN 50 WORDS IN PART II OF THE PAPER.

*August 1975*

**Central Midwives Board for Scotland**

EXAMINATION PAPER I

*From 10.30 a.m. to 12.30 p.m.*

*Candidates should answer ALL FOUR Questions*

1. Describe the anatomy of the Fallopian tube. What abnormalities of the tube may interfere with fertilisation and/or embedding of the ovum?
2. Describe in detail the admission procedure of a patient in labour.
3. Describe the management of a patient with vaginal bleeding re-admitted to hospital 12 days after delivery.
4. What is/are:
   (a) Decidual reaction
   (b) Amniocentesis
   (c) Oestrogens
   (d) Engagement of the fetal head
   (e) Deep transverse arrest?

*August 1975*

**Central Midwives Board for Scotland**

EXAMINATION PAPER II

*From 2.00 p.m. to 4.00 p.m.*

*Candidates should answer ALL FOUR Questions*

1. Give a detailed description of the routine examination of a newborn baby.
2. What are the causes of vomiting in the first week of life? Describe the investigation and management.
3. Describe the content of talks, given during the antenatal period, dealing with:
   (a) Diet

    (b) Clothing
    (c) Smoking
4. What is/are:
    (a) Infant mortality
    (b) Registration of stillbirths
    (c) Family allowance
    (d) Adoption
    (e) Non-accidental injury in a child?

## The Northern Ireland Council for Nurses and Midwives

### EXAMINATION FOR STUDENT MIDWIVES

*Wednesday 1st October 1975*    *From 10.00 a.m. to 1.00 p.m.*

*Candidates MUST attempt ALL questions*

1. Describe the fetal skull and the changes that occur in it during labour.
2. Define antepartum haemorrhage and enumerate its causes. Describe the initial management of a patient admitted with bleeding per vaginam at the 34th week of pregnancy.
3. What are the indications for induction of labour? What are the dangers associated with induction and indicate the precautions which should be taken to avoid complications.
4. Describe the management of a baby who fails to breathe at birth.
5. Describe the special problems related to unmarried women. What services are available to her before and after delivery?
6. Write short notes on *five* of the following:
    (a) Döderlein's bacillus
    (b) Alpha-fetoprotein
    (c) The 'safe' period
    (d) External cephalic version
    (e) Ergometrine (oxytocic agents)
    (f) Involution
    (g) Postnatal clinics
    (h) 'Late deceleration'

Many similarities are to be noted in the format of these papers. Six questions are to be answered in three hours: four in two hours. Clearly 30 minutes is a standard time for answering one question. Questions needing short answers occur more frequently, particularly in the English papers, where it seems reasonable to infer that one 'long' question is equivalent to four 'short' ones. An average 'short' answer may thus be compiled in seven or eight minutes.

Nor is there any appreciable choice. One such concession occurs in Part I of the Community Health paper, in which two out of three questions are to be answered in one hour; while in the Northern Ireland paper the candidate is to write short notes on five out of a choice of eight subjects.

The subjects are, by tradition, pigeon-holed, albeit approximately: anatomy/physiology; pregnancy; labour; puerperium; the newborn child; and community health. A study of the examination papers above will show how the range of questions extends over these subjects; none is omitted. Paediatrics and community care receive special emphasis, in line with current thought.

It is obvious from the outset that careful training in answering questions is necessary; the best way that a candidate can prepare herself in this respect is by making herself plan and write an answer to a given question in the space of half an hour. Those candidates who are conscious of slowness of any kind, in thinking, planning, or writing, arc particularly recommended to practise in this way.

Although it is, of course, the material in an examination answer which gains the marks, the style is not without influence on the examiner.

The script that is legibly written and neatly set out, with the correct headings numbered and, where necessary, underlined, will immediately produce a favourable impression. On the other hand, untidy and barely legible writing, the smudgy 'carbon copy' effect of some ball-point pens, and lack of paragraphing or other obvious emphasis cannot but impress any examiner unfavourably.

If an answer is written in good English and accurately punctuated, its meaning is immediately clear. An ungrammatical and unpunctuated account, however excellent the subject matter, is much more difficult to understand; and sometimes the careless construction of a sentence will completely distort its meaning.

Spelling is more important than is sometimes realized. Probably the majority of examiners would not quibble about an occasional spelling mistake; but repeated mis-spelling of words in common use creates, reasonably enough, an impression of carelessness. Moreover, it could be argued that a candidate who is careless, or inattentive to detail in one respect may well behave in the same way in other circumstances.

Many candidates feel that they could write a much better examination paper if there were no time limit. It is very natural that an overseas candidate, who is writing the paper in a foreign language, should be conscious of this difficulty; nor is it confined to those students with language problems. The not very quick thinkers and the slow writers are at a disadvantage. So, too, are those nervous candidates who remain for the first half-hour in a paralytic state, and only after this accustom themselves to the climate of the examination room.

Probably the best way of easing this difficulty, if the cause of the trouble cannot be removed, is to plan the answer so that there is less to write; and there are a few ways in which this can be achieved.

It is useful to practise beforehand picking out the essential points which must be included in an answer, and concentrating on these: if necessary, to the exclusion of the more unlikely contingencies. In the question, for example, of postpartum haemorrhage of unspecified source, bleeding from the placental site, during or just after the third stage of labour must be included, as fully as possible; to omit this would be inexcusable. Traumatic haemorrhage, on the other hand, might be excluded, or briefly mentioned without any great loss of marks. Similarly, in the management of twin labour, an oblique lie of the second child is always a possibility; twin locking is so highly improbable as hardly to be worth mentioning.

An answer which is correctly tabulated is likely to be more concise than one which is written in essay form. But, while tabulation is permissible, and often desirable, its meaning must be clearly understood. It means planning and setting out the answer using a series of headings; in some cases each may have its own sequence of sub-headings. It does not mean writing an answer in the telegraphic style which is used for note-taking, omitting all definite and indefinite articles, and many adjectives and verbs. Nor does it mean indiscriminate abbreviation, which is indefensible. This is not to suggest that the script should be written in any very elaborate or fancy style; nor is the polished English of the essayist a necessity. Short, simple sentences which are correctly punctuated are usually clear in their meaning and implication; and this is enough.

The planning of the sequences also needs care. A list, e.g., of a dozen 'causes' of pyrexia in the postnatal period, without explanation, can be repetitive and incorrect, thus:

(a) retained products of conception
(b) infection of the genital tract
(c) urinary tract infection, pyelonephritis
(d) infection of perineal lacerations
(e) infection of the placental site
(f) infection of breast, breast abscess
(g) cystitis
(h) mastitis
(i) puerperal sepsis, etc.

This is an obvious and glaring example of all that is worst in faulty tabulation. It is considered in detail here because it is one of the commonest weaknesses seen in examination scripts; and the appalling sequence above is not as much exaggerated as might be supposed. This muddled list should, of course, read:

(a) urinary tract infection
    (i) cystitis
    (ii) pyelonephritis
(b) genital tract infection (puerperal sepsis)
    (i) infection of the placental site
    (ii) infection of perineal lacerations
(c) breast infection
    (i) mastitis
    (ii) breast abscess

Note that retained products of conception are not a cause of pyrexia; they may easily become infected, and the bacterial infection causes the pyrexia.

Diagrams can be valuable time-savers. A simple diagram, provided it be clear and accurately labelled, can explain adequately not only the structure of a particular organ, but its anatomical relationships, which might otherwise need two or three pages of script.

Such a diagram saves not only the candidate's but the examiner's time, as does any kind of chart, graph, or tracing: always with the proviso that it be accurately reproduced. That overworked cliché 'everything can be seen at a glance' is so true of most simple diagrams and charts that it should be kept constantly in mind by candidates writing examination answers.

Diagrams can be used to particular advantage by those overseas students who find difficulty in writing English quickly. A clear picture can illustrate many points and supersedes all language barriers; and, moreover, much time that might have been spent on a written explanation is saved.

All diagrams should be sufficiently large. At least half a page should be allowed; a whole page should be used if necessary, and marginal thumb-nail sketches should be avoided at all costs.

Colour is a great asset in diagrams, and all candidates are advised to bring a few coloured crayons or fibre pens to the examination. Such subjects as the blood supply to the uterus, the fetal circulation, and antepartum haemorrhage can be illustrated in black and white only with the greatest difficulty and with some risk of confusion. Red and blue crayons, however, can be used to illustrate these details quickly and clearly.

One of the most important aspects of an examination answer is its relevance. It is as essential as accuracy and, indeed, irrelevance *is* inaccuracy: in that, if a statement, however true in itself, is irrelevant as an answer to a certain question, then it is an inaccurate answer to that question.

Many marks are lost unnecessarily through irrelevance. In some cases, most of the answer is correct, but some irrelevant material is introduced. This is quite likely to happen when the candidate has a good knowledge of the subject; in her enthusiasm she may write down everything she knows about the subject, relevant or not. It would be easy, for instance, in discussing the causes of delay in the second stage of labour, to include diagnosis or treatment, as well as causes; but it would not be relevant.

Sometimes, however, the candidate misinterprets the entire question, and writes a wholly irrelevant account, without answering the question at all. Candidates set a question about antepartum haemorrhage have been known to write only about postpartum haemorrhage. This may sound absurd; and, indeed, perhaps outside the examination room, it is. But, in the mental turmoil which the examination evokes in some candidates, it is all too possible.

It is obviously desirable to try to avoid this common error. The candidate is therefore advised to read and re-read the question frequently: before writing any notes at all: before re-arranging the notes into an orderly outline: and before, during and after the final writing of the answer. On each occasion the candidate should ask herself: 'Is this all relevant?'

The examination papers, ranging as they do over a variety of subjects, yet conform fairly closely to an orthodox order. One question may well deal with anatomy and/or physiology, almost always with some practical application. Other questions are on pregnancy, labour, the infant and, possibly, the postnatal period, sometimes actually in this order.

The order in which these questions are answered is a matter for consideration. All must be answered and on no account should a candidate risk leaving a question totally unanswered, however little she knows of the subject. Since there is no choice, there is much to be said for the practice of beginning with the first question and working straight through the paper to the end. Certainly it is wise to tackle the more demanding questions fairly early, when the mind is fresh; and those candidates who experience difficulty in learning anatomy and physiology should never be tempted to shelve a question on this subject until the last half-hour. Anyone who has sat through a long written examination is familiar with the state of mental exhaustion that is appreciated to the full only after the ordeal is over. This weariness has, of course, been building up gradually and, clearly half an hour before the end is not the best moment to approach the most exacting question on the paper. It is inescapable that the more difficult questions should be answered earlier.

On the other hand, it may be extremely foolhardy to answer the 'short notes' type of question first, since, given *carte blanche* – short notes on any aspect of the subject – it is all too tempting to write, not brief notes, but quite a long account; and, indeed, to over-run the time allowance. Conversely, the candidate who *has* over-run her time and has only twenty minutes in which to answer her last question and read through her script can probably cope adequately with this type of answer – and this type only – in the few minutes remaining. Thus, however this question paper is viewed, it seems sensible to begin at the beginning and go straight through to the end. Most examiners, too, probably prefer marking in this order. Indeed, to an examiner, marking steadily through a pile of scripts, nine orderly and straightforward, the tenth, with its grasshopper-like approach to the questions, can prove very disconcerting and more time-consuming.

In the oral examination, the candidate meets two examiners: one, an obstetrician and the other, a midwife. Both have marked her script. The examiners may or may not make reference to the paper; certainly the candidate should be prepared for such a reference, which may give her a good opportunity to fill an omission or to correct an error. Thus, while the common post-examination practice of conducting an autopsy on the paper may seem unnecessarily morbid and can indeed be depressing; yet, taken in a constructive way, it may prove a most salutary exercise and is not to be condemned out of hand. It is always better to be aware of one's errors than completely to disregard them.

Whenever two categories of person meet on common ground a 'we' and 'they' situation is apt to develop. Nowhere is the distinction between 'us' and 'them' more sharply defined than between examinees and examiners. Some candidates accept this relationship, thriving in a healthy atmosphere of genial antagonism; others, lacking this assurance, see only the differences and divisions, losing sight of the common aim. This is a matter for regret to examiners.

The situation develops in the oral examination. 'I didn't know what they were getting at.' 'It was so simple; they must have been trying to catch me out.' Worst of all, the damnatory faint praise of 'They were very nice (kind/understanding/pleasant/patient) but. . . .'

It needs to be stated categorically and stressed frequently that examiners and candidates are all on the same side. They meet with a common objective: to pass the examination. The candidate knows that she herself wants to pass. It seems sometimes to escape her that the examiners want to pass her. If only she gives them the opportunity they will do so gladly. Examiners are obstetricians and midwives, working in maternity units where good midwives are wanted. And when the rather despondent candidate leaves the examination room, perhaps it is a pity that she cannot hear 'their' remarks. The midwife: 'I'd like her in the labour ward,' and the obstetrician's high praise: 'I wouldn't mind her looking after my wife.'

# Diagrams

# Diagrams

## A SAGITTAL SECTION OF THE PELVIS

A diagrammatic sagittal section of the female pelvis has many uses. It is a little more ambitious than the simple square or circle type of diagram, but it is not really difficult to draw. A little practice is needed and, indeed, is valuable as an aid to anatomical study, in that the size and relationship of the pelvic bones and organs must be kept constantly in mind.

This diagram [Fig. 1(a)], or part of it, may be used to illustrate a wide range of subjects, of which the planes of the pelvis; the anatomy of the bladder; engagement of the presenting part; the

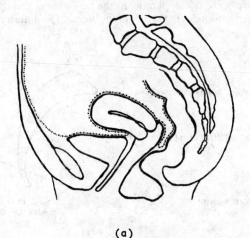

**(a)**

FIG. 1(a). A simplified sagittal section of the pelvis

vagina and its anatomical relations; and the non-pregnant uterus may be quoted as a few examples.

The symphysis pubis should be drawn first, at an angle of about 35° to the horizontal. It is 3·5 cm deep, and from this the scale of the diagram can be kept in mind.

From the uppermost point of the symphysis pubis a guide-line AB is drawn at an angle of 55° to the horizontal. A similar line, CD, is drawn at an angle of 15°, from the lower border of the symphysis. See Fig. 1(b). These lines represent the planes of the pelvic brim and outlet, respectively, and, depending on the purpose of the diagram, they may be retained, or rubbed out later.

The sacral promontory is marked on AB, 11 cm from A, i.e. 3 times the depth of the symphysis. The lower border of the sacrum is marked on CD, 13 cm away, or 3½ times the depth of the symphysis. A curved line joining these two points is the anterior surface of the sacrum. It is not difficult now to add the posterior surface, the fifth lumbar vertebra and the coccyx.

The uterus, about twice the depth of the symphysis pubis, lies in the centre of the pelvic cavity, in an anteverted attitude. The vaginal walls are drawn parallel to the pelvic brim, and approximately at right-angles to the axis of the uterus. The anterior wall is

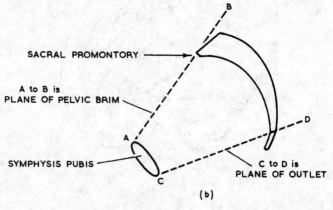

**(b)**

FIG. 1(b). Diagram to show the pelvis in sagittal section

the same depth as the uterus, the posterior wall one-third greater.
See Fig. 1(c).

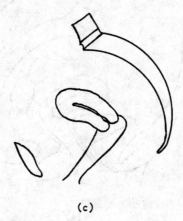

(c)

The bladder occupies the space behind the symphysis pubis. Its
base is related to the anterior vaginal wall and the cervix. The

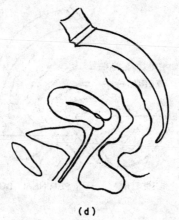

(d)

FIG. 1, (c) and (d). Diagrams to show the pelvis in sagittal section

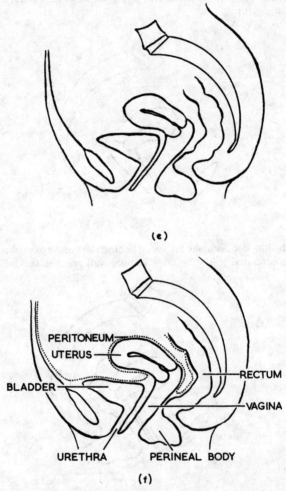

FIG. 1, (e) and (f). Diagrams to show the pelvis in sagittal section

urethra, 3·5 cm long, lies very close to the anterior vaginal wall.

The rectum lies behind the uterus and vagina, the pouch of Douglas separating it from the uppermost third of the vagina. It lies in close contact with the middle third and then turns sharply backwards to terminate in the anal canal, separated from the lowest third of the posterior vaginal wall by the perineal body. See Fig. 1(d).

A single line is sufficient to represent the superficial structures, e.g. abdominal wall, thigh, etc. See Fig. 1(e).

The pelvic peritoneum is now added, the uterovesical pouch reaching to the isthmus of the uterus, and the pouch of Douglas extending well behind the posterior vaginal fornix. The line should be clearly distinguishable, and preferably drawn in another colour. The relevant structures should then be clearly labelled. See Fig. 1(f). The indicating lines, where possible, should be parallel.


## THE SHAPE OF THE PELVIS

The bony pelvis is not easy to reproduce accurately without considerable practice; pictures of the pelvic girdle are better avoided by all but the most competent artists.

On the other hand, the shape of the pelvis – brim, cavity and outlet – can be adequately illustrated by means of simple outlines.

The brim is slightly ovoid, with the sacral promontory projecting forwards. It may be easier to begin with a complete circle, and then to draw in the posterior boundary of the brim. See Fig. 2(a).

The pelvis at mid-cavity level may be shown as a circle, without alteration. If compasses are used, no freehand drawing is necessary. See Fig. 2(b).

The outlet is diamond-shaped, or slightly ovoid, and the four straight lines, or two arcs which represent it are quickly drawn. See Fig. 2(c).

The diameters should be drawn in contrasting colours.

The depth of the cavity may be shown by drawing the symphysis pubis and the sacrum and coccyx in sagittal section, as in Fig. 1(b), page 28.

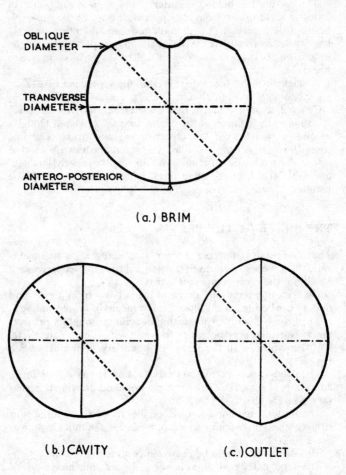

(a.) BRIM

(b.) CAVITY

(c.) OUTLET

FIG. 2. The shape of the pelvis

## THE FETAL SKULL

Most candidates will find it difficult – if not impossible – to draw an adequate diagram of the fetal skull, with all its intricate bones. Yet this diagram can be useful to illustrate diameters, moulding and the various swellings which may be seen on the child's head.

There are two alternatives:

1. To draw an outline of the skull; all detail of the facial and other bones, except perhaps rough indications of the cranial bones and the orbit, is omitted. This is not particularly difficult. The outline fits into a rectangle having a depth of seven-eighths of its width, e.g. 7 cm × 8 cm or 3½ in × 4 in. This can be drawn in pencil and afterwards rubbed out. See Fig. 3.

2. To draw two curved lines, representing the shape of the child's head, with the soft tissues. This is easier, and sufficient to illustrate

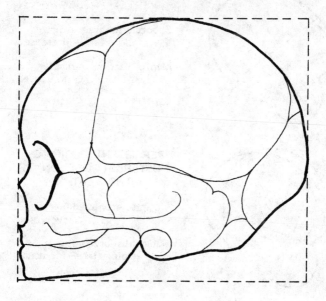

FIG. 3. Outline of the fetal skull

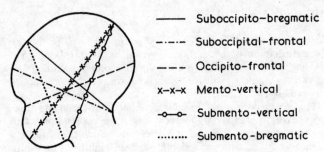

— Suboccipito-bregmatic
-·-·- Suboccipital-frontal
--- Occipito-frontal
x-x-x Mento-vertical
-o—o- Submento-vertical
........ Submento-bregmatic

FIG. 4. Longitudinal diameters of the fetal skull

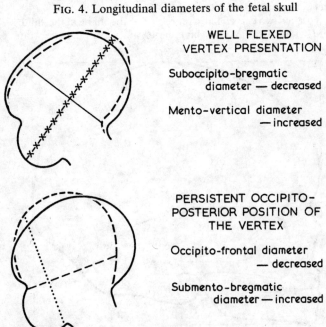

WELL FLEXED
VERTEX PRESENTATION

Suboccipito-bregmatic
    diameter — decreased

Mento-vertical diameter
                — increased

PERSISTENT OCCIPITO-
POSTERIOR POSITION OF
THE VERTEX

Occipito-frontal diameter
                — decreased

Submento-bregmatic
    diameter — increased

FIG. 5. Moulding of the fetal skull

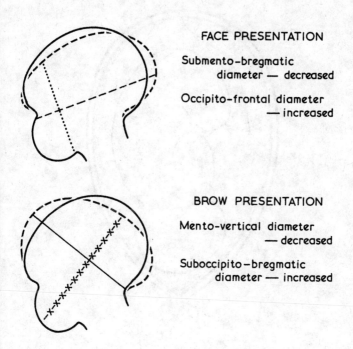

FACE PRESENTATION

Submento-bregmatic
        diameter — decreased

Occipito-frontal diameter
             — increased

BROW PRESENTATION

Mento-vertical diameter
             — decreased

Suboccipito-bregmatic
        diameter — increased

FIG. 5 (contd). Moulding of the fetal skull

most answers of this type. See Fig. 4, Longitudinal diameters of
the fetal skull, and Fig. 5, Moulding of the fetal skull.

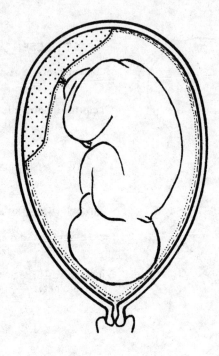

Fig. 6. The fetus in utero

This is useful to illustrate a variety of subjects.

It will be found easier to draw the uterus first, and then to fit the fetus into it. It is satisfactory to divide the uterus into three equal parts and to begin by drawing the fetal head, making it occupy the whole of the lowest third. Then the trunk and limbs are drawn. A simple outline is just as effective as an elaborately shaded picture. The placenta and chorion should be in the same colour; the amnion in a contrasting colour.

## PLACENTA PRAEVIA

Placenta praevia is not difficult to illustrate, but, again, colours are necessary. It is much clearer and little more trouble to show the different types on separate pictures. When they are superimposed the effect can be rather confused; and, in most cases, simple diagrams are preferable to complex ones. See Fig. 7.

Proportions are important. The uterus at term measures 30–35 cm from fundus to cervix. The placenta is about 20 cm in diameter. (The fetal dolls, used in teaching midwifery, are frequently made with their placentae absurdly small, and this tendency is sometimes seen in diagrams.) The lower uterine segment, as nearly as can be stated, is the lowermost one-quarter, or rather less, of the uterus.

The uterus may be shown as a single thick line, preferably in a neutral colour, such as brown. The placenta is best in purple, or perhaps blue, and can be drawn partially separated from the uterine wall, with a trickle of blood (red) showing in clear contrast.

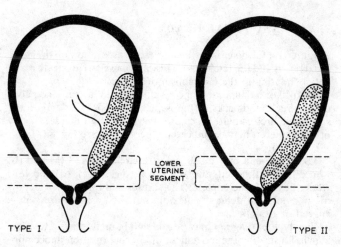

LOWER
UTERINE
SEGMENT

TYPE I                                                   TYPE II

FIG. 7. Placenta Praevia

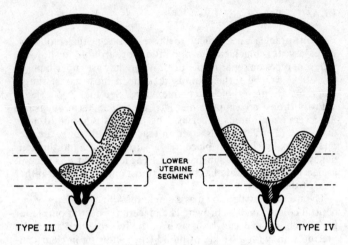

Fig. 7 (contd.). Placenta Praevia

## PELVIS AND FETAL HEAD

Another useful diagram is a simple representation of the maternal pelvis and the fetal head. This can be used to illustrate many details relating to the mechanism of labour.

An oval or a diamond shape is sufficient to illustrate the pelvic outlet. Such landmarks as the ischial tuberosities or spines and sub-pubic arch should be clearly marked. The oblique, or any other diameter, may be indicated if necessary. See Fig. 8 (a), (b), (c), (d), (e).

The fetal head may be shown as a circle (Figs. 8 (a) and (b) where it is well flexed, and as an oval (Figs. 8 (c), (d) and (e) ) where flexion is incomplete. The sutures and fontanelles, denoting not only the degree of flexion, but the position, are simply curved or straight lines.

This type of diagram may be adapted in many ways. Here it is shown illustrating the movement of internal rotation in occipito-anterior position. Persistent occipito-posterior position and deep

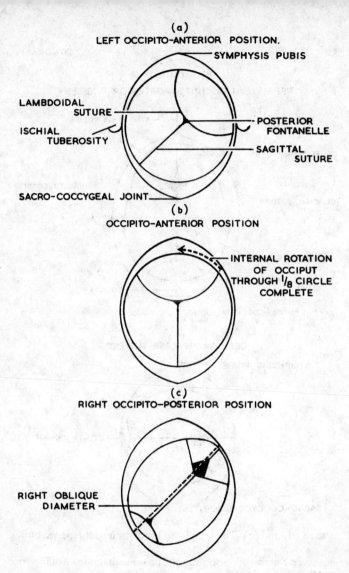

FIG. 8, (a), (b) and (c). The fetal head in relation to the pelvic outlet

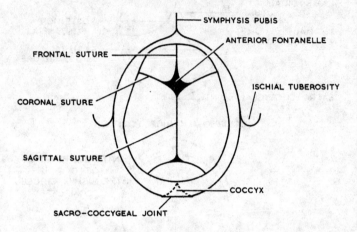

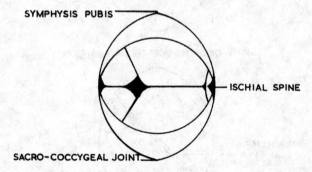

FIG. 8 (d) and (e). The fetal head in relation to the pelvic outlet

transverse arrest are also shown. The same diagrams would serve
to illustrate the findings on vaginal examination.

## GRAPHS

Another type of diagram is the graph. Graphs and diagrammatic charts are used increasingly in patients' case notes where they have the great advantage that a number of related factors can be seen at a glance. Not only does this save time, but the relationships are immediately obvious and accurate assessment is easier. The simplest example of all is the rising pulse rate and falling blood pressure in haemorrhage. The graph of temperature, pulse and respiration is another simple example. The partograph (Fig. 9) and the Apgar score (see Q. 208, p. 191) are similarly useful, particularly if marked according to the hospital pattern.

Graphs are equally valuable in examinations. With a little practice they are soon drawn and they quickly convey a great deal of information: in this case, to the examiner, who is an obstetrician or a midwife well accustomed to reading graphs. They reduce the amount of writing and thus save the candidate's precious time (and the examiner's in marking). Babies' weight curves, mortality rates, pre-eclampsia charts, urinary oestriol excretion rates related to weeks of pregnancy and fluid balance records are only a few examples of their many uses.

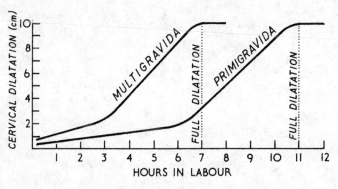

Fig. 9. Partograph

# Anatomy and Physiology

# Anatomy and Physiology

**Q.1. Describe the female bladder and urethra.**
**Give the obstetrical causes of retention of urine.**

Since the description of the bladder and urethra in this answer may represent fifteen or twenty minutes' work, it is clear that no very minute detail is expected; it is sufficient to present the gross anatomy, and to consider structure quite briefly.

The anatomical facts should be given in an orderly sequence, and it is usually convenient to tabulate these facts.

A clear and accurate diagram, however simple, is a valuable addition. It may save a good deal of writing and it is often useful in presenting the subject matter in a concise way. Part of Fig. 1 may be used, suitably enlarged.

The second part of the question does not require a greatly detailed answer; the remaining ten minutes should allow enough time to cover this.

It should be borne in mind that lack of knowledge of anatomy and, therefore, a brief, sketchy, and incomplete answer, cannot be compensated by 'padding' in the second part of the answer.

Finally, it is important to remember that, though brief and simple, this part of the question is of great practical importance as a responsibility of the midwife.

**Answer.** The female bladder and urethra.

### The Bladder
1. *General* characteristics: a hollow muscular organ situated in the pelvic cavity and acting as a reservoir of urine.
2. *Shape:* approximately pyramidal, with the apex directed forwards.
3. *Capacity:* normally up to 500 ml; exceptionally, much more.

4. *Relations:*

(a) anteriorly: the pubes and the symphysis: retro-pubic fat.

(b) posteriorly: the cervix and upper anterior vaginal wall.

(c) superiorly: the utero-vesical pouch of peritoneum and the fundus uteri.

(d) inferiorly: the triangular ligament.

(e) laterally: the retro-pubic fat and the levatores ani.

Within the bladder, at the base, three orifices form the angles of a triangular area termed the trigone. These are the two ureters, entering laterally, and the urethra, a narrow canal 3·5–4 cm long, leaving centrally.

5. *Blood supply:* from the superior and inferior vesical arteries, from the internal iliac arteries. The venous drainage is similar.

6. *Structure:* four layers:

A. Peritoneum: covers the superior aspect only.

B. Muscle: three muscle layers; outer longitudinal, middle circular, and inner longitudinal fibres. This muscle, which contracts to empty the bladder, is known as the detrusor muscle.

C. Sub-mucous layer; the sub-mucosa is very loosely attached to the muscle.

D. Mucous membrane: this, with the exception of the area of the trigone, is thrown into folds when the bladder is empty. The lining is of transitional epithelium.

## The Urethra

The urethra is a narrow tube leading from the internal meatus to the vestibule. It lies almost embedded in the lower half of the anterior vaginal wall. Where it leaves the bladder (the bladder neck) is a thick band of circular muscle forming the internal sphincter. Nearer the vestibule is the so-called external sphincter, which has a compressing rather than a constricting action.

*Blood supply:* From the inferior vesical and pudendal arteries. The venous return is similar.

*Structure:* three layers.

Muscle: an outer circular layer of smooth muscle and an inner longitudinal layer, continuous with that lining the bladder.

A vascular layer of connective tissue.

A lining, in the upper half, of transitional epithelium, as in the bladder and in the lower half, of squamous epithelium.

*Function.* The bladder and urethra work in harmony. The bladder acts as a reservoir for urine, the walls stretching as it fills, while the urethral sphincters remain contracted to prevent the escape of urine.

In voiding, this action is reversed. The sphincters relax, the detrusor muscle contracts and, aided by an increase of intra-abdominal pressure, the bladder is emptied.

### Obstetrical causes of retention of urine

In pregnancy, it is uncommon. Acute urinary retention may arise at the 14th or 15th week, if a retroverted gravid uterus should become incarcerated below the sacral promontory.

In labour, retention is common in the late first stage and in the second stage as, with the stretching of the anterior vaginal wall, the urethra becomes increasingly elongated and narrowed; eventually voiding may be impossible.

In the puerperium, retention of urine is not uncommon, especially in patients who remain entirely in bed for twenty-four hours after delivery. Many simple factors can contribute to it: abnormal posture, unaccustomedness to the use of a bedpan, lack of privacy; pain from local trauma or oedema; fear of pain, of straining, or of breaking sutures; and lack of awareness that the bladder is distended.

Urinary retention may be complete or partial, the retention of residual amounts of urine being the more serious, since it can be overlooked. This increases the risk that the urine may become infected and can also lead to retention with overflow.

**Q.2. Describe the anatomy of the bladder. How may urinary infections be avoided in pregnancy, labour and puerperium?**

The first part of this question is exactly the same as the preceding one. The second part is simple, straightforward and practical.

Question 3, below, includes much of the practical features of Question 1 and Question 2, but no actual anatomy.

**Q.3. What are the indications for catheterization of the bladder in the obstetric patient?** *(Scotland)*

**Q.4. Describe the urinary bladder.**
**What abnormalities of micturition may occur in pregnancy, labour and puerperium?**

This is similar to Q.1, but with two differences:
1. The urethra is not mentioned. It cannot, however, be omitted from the answer. Indeed, exactly the same description as in the answer to Q.1. would be perfectly appropriate. Physiologically, the urethra functions with the bladder. In our practical care and observation of patients, we bracket the urethra with the bladder. Similarly, many experts, setting examination questions think of 'bladder' as 'bladder and urethra', 'placenta' as 'placenta and membranes' and 'fetal skull' as 'fetal skull and scalp' and, perhaps, even 'intracranial contents'.
2. 'Abnormalities of micturition' is more than 'retention of urine', but does not include all complications involving the urinary tract. Increased frequency of micturition (when it is abnormal) and urinary incontinence in all its manifestations are relevant. So is dysuria; but not oliguria. Urinary tract infection is relevant only in so far as it may give rise to dysuria and increased frequency.

**Q.5. What changes occur in the urinary tract during pregnancy? Give the management of a patient with acute pyelonephritis.** *(Scotland)*

A straightforward question, requiring, first, an orderly account of the changes in the urinary tract in normal pregnancy. This might well end with the kinking and dilatation of the ureters which favours the development of urinary tract infection.

Secondly, a fairly abrupt change to the management of a patient who has acute pyelonephritis. Straightforward enough, again, but the key-word 'management' must be kept in mind. Management means medical and nursing care and observation. The midwife (as she hopes soon to be) must know the records the doctor will wish to see, the treatment that he will recommend and the drugs, with their dosage, that he is likely to prescribe. All this can be stated briefly, so that time is left to include the nursing care (the midwife's job) in rather more detail. Both obstetrician and midwife examiner will commend the candidate who shows a sense of proportion between her own work and that of her medical colleague.

**Q.6. How may the urinary tract be affected by pregnancy and labour?**

Here the basic physiology and anatomy are again taken for granted and the candidate is invited to spend her full quota of examination time, 30 minutes, on a broader issue: namely, how the whole of the urinary tract – not only the bladder – may be affected by pregnancy and labour. There is a need to include normal changes, proceeding then through the common disorders such as asymptomatic bacteriuria and glycosuria to a short consideration of the more serious abnormalities.

**Q.7. Describe the functions of the placenta. What may give rise to impairment of these functions?**

This is one example of a fairly common type of anatomy and physiology question. As usual, the question, though primarily theoretical, has a clear practical significance. Here, there is a good deal to be said about impairment of functions. The account of the function of the placenta might therefore represent only about one half of the answer. On the other hand, 'describe' rather than 'outline' implies that some detail is necessary and a bare list of functions would be insufficient.

**Answer.** The functions of the placenta may be described thus:

1. *Respiration.* The placenta is the organ whereby oxygen from the maternal blood is passed to the fetal blood, and whereby carbon dioxide resulting from fetal metabolism is returned to the

maternal blood for excretion.

2. *Nutrition.* It is via the placenta that foodstuffs, mineral salts and vitamins necessary to the growth and development of the fetus pass from the mother's to the child's blood.

3. *Excretion.* As well as carbon dioxide, other waste products of metabolism are passed by the placenta from the fetal to the maternal blood for excretion.

4. *Protection.* The so-called barrier function of the placenta is a partial protection only to the child. Some bacteria, antibodies, drugs, etc., can pass the placental barrier; others cannot. Examples of such bacteria are the tubercle bacillus, which may circulate in the mother's blood, but which practically never gains entrance to the fetal blood; and the spirochaete of syphilis, which does pass the placental barrier. A woman with untreated syphilis will therefore give birth to a syphilitic child.

5. *Hormone production.* From the second week of pregnancy the primitive trophoblastic tissue is elaborating chorionic gonadotrophin. This continues throughout the pregnancy. By the twelfth week of pregnancy, the placenta is fully formed, and from then onwards it produces other hormones. Hitherto these have been secreted by the anterior lobe of the pituitary gland and the corpus luteum of the ovary. Now the corpus luteum degenerates and the placenta secretes oestrogens and progesterone. In this way, the placenta not only supports the pregnancy, allowing the steady growth of the uterus, and maintaining a healthy lining within it, but prepares the breasts and nipples for lactation.

The functions of the placenta may become impaired as a result of any of the following developments:

**In pregnancy:**

1. *Premature separation of the placenta,* whether it is situated normally (abruptio placentae) or abnormally (placenta praevia). If one-third or more of the placenta becomes separated it is extremely improbable that the fetus will survive.

2. *Pre-eclampsia,* with development of areas of infarcted, and therefore functionless placental tissue.

3. *Antenatal eclampsia,* which is rare, but particularly dangerous in that the already impaired placental function is aggravated by

the apnoeic phase of the mother's eclamptic fit.

4. *Essential hypertension.*

5. *Chronic renal disease.*

In these last two conditions, the placental function may be impaired in a manner similar to that in pre-eclampsia. Furthermore, any one of these three conditions may be associated with abruptio placentae.

6. *Heavy smoking* has been shown to retard placental and fetal growth.

7. *Prolongation of pregnancy.* The placenta's activity gradually decreases in the last few weeks of pregnancy. At the 41st week it is slightly less than at term and after the 42nd week the fetus is appreciably at risk from a placental insufficiency that will be worsened by the uterine contractions as labour advances.

Sometimes placental insufficiency cannot be accounted for.

**In Labour:**

1. The contractions of normal labour will naturally worsen any pre-existing placental insufficiency.

2. *Early rupture of the membranes* with great loss of liquor amnii may lead to compression of the placenta, with some interference with its functions.

3. *Twin labour.* After the birth of the first child, the uterus is much smaller, the placental site smaller and the oxygen supply to the second twin decreased. Thus a second twin is at greater risk than the first.

4. *Any accident of labour* involving placenta or cord, such as cord prolapse may render the placenta completely functionless.

The first part of Q.8 is similar.

**Q.8. Describe: (a) the functions of the placenta; (b) the normal placenta after delivery.**

**State the Central Midwives Board for Scotland rules regarding the placenta.** *(Scotland)*

The second part is even simpler than that of Q.7: a description of the placenta after delivery. Here, there are two factors to be borne in mind. Firstly, in describing the placenta, the candidate should have in her mind, not the textbook, nor the classroom, but the labour ward; it is the placenta that she has seen examined and herself examined so often that is to be described; and in recalling the procedure she will have a ready-made orderly account to present. Secondly, the over-cautious candidate, perhaps intimidated by the examination room atmosphere, may ask herself: 'Do I include the membranes and cord? They're not mentioned.' The answer to this lies also in the labour ward and the midwife, who is saying, 'Well, now, are you ready to examine the placenta?' Clearly the membranes and the cord are to be included, whether in the delivery room or in the examination.

Q.9, again, begins similarly:

## Q.9. Describe the functions of the placenta. How may placental function be assessed? *(Scotland)*

The second part of this question should be read and re-read carefully with attention to its precise meaning. It is rather broader than merely placental function tests. These, of course, should be included; but it is worth while mentioning also the various modes of measuring fetal growth, since this is not simply related to, but actually dependent on placental function.

## Q.10. Describe the functions of the placenta. How may the efficiency of the placenta be impaired?

This question is almost precisely similar to Question 7.

## Q.11. Give a detailed description of the normal placenta at term. Enumerate its functions. *(Scotland)*

In answering this question, much more time should be allocated to the first part of the answer. The placental functions can be enumerated in a very few minutes.

**Q.12. Describe the functions of the placenta. Why are the placenta and membranes examined after delivery?**

Placental function is a matter of immediate interest to the midwife. In the labour ward she sees and examines placentae every day. She has every opportunity to compare a placenta with the baby who was supported by it as a fetus in utero. Not surprisingly, this is a fairly common examination subject. It is true that the placenta is now appreciated to be a very highly complex organ, having elaborate functions which are only beginning to be understood. How much physiology should a midwife know? The upper limit is probably to be determined by her own interest. The minimum may be defined as enough to do her work intelligently and responsibly. This includes understanding the functions of the placenta at a fairly basic level.

The second part of the answer is largely a recollection of day-to-day routines, which are then to be explained.

Finally, the candidate is enjoined to read the question carefully and to answer what has been asked. For some unexplained reason this type of question comes across to the occasional candidate as 'How?' and not 'Why?' The experts who drafted the question surely feel that after six months or more of midwifery training the candidate is sufficiently well versed in the actual procedure, but that it may be desirable to determine whether she understands its purpose.

The first part of this answer is set out in the answer to Q.7. The second part is below.

**Answer.** As soon as possible after delivery, the placenta and membranes are examined for a variety of reasons.

The most urgent need is to ascertain whether or not the placenta and membranes are complete. Retained placental tissue, even a fragment, is dangerous. It prevents effective contraction and retraction of the uterus and, sooner or later, secondary post-partum haemorrhage, sometimes of serious degree, will occur. Furthermore, this necrotic tissue favours the growth of pathogens and thus predisposes to puerperal infection. Retained chorion is troublesome rather than dangerous, in that it may be associated with rather profuse and offensive lochia and sub-involution.

It is interesting to compare the size and weight of the placenta with that of the infant, noting also the period of gestation. The large healthy vascular placenta and the well-nourished baby are in striking contrast to the small, avascular, infarcted placenta and the puny small-for-dates child. Similarly the calcified placenta in postmaturity.

Other anomalies and abnormalities may be revealed by careful examination, yielding valuable information. Examples are the blood vessels leading to a hole in the membranes, denoting the retention of a succenturiate lobe; and the cord having only two vessels, which suggests a renal abnormality in the child.

Following twin delivery of infants of the same sex, the membranes can show whether the infants are monozygotic or dizygotic twins.

**Q.13. Give a brief description of the placenta at term. What are its functions?** *(Northern Ireland)*

Here is a question very similar to Question 11, but with a marked change of emphasis and obviously needing a more elaborate account of the placental functions.

**Q.14. Describe the structure of the placenta. What abnormalities may occur?** *(Scotland)*

Quite a different type of question. In Question 13, structure is not required; here, it is. Again, more time should be allocated for the first part of the answer than the second, though the term 'abnormalities' gives the candidate much scope.

**Q.15. What are the functions of the placenta? How may placental function be monitored in pregnancy?**

This question, very similar to Questions 7 and 10, only serves to underline the importance of this very essential aspect of antenatal care. The candidate will best answer this question by reviewing her experience in the antenatal clinics and wards recalling the patients who were submitted to so many tests, and assessing the babies born to these patients.

**Q.16. Describe the methods available for monitoring the fetus during pregnancy and labour.** *(Scotland)*

This question is included here because it illustrates so well the more oblique approach to physiology which is characteristic of present-day examination questions. The candidate must know her physiology; she must also know how to apply it.

These last two questions are placed together as a reminder of a fact that is still sometimes lost sight of: that the fetus and the placenta are one single organism.

**Q.17. Describe the vagina. What information may be obtained from a vaginal examination during labour?**

It is not surprising that questions about the vagina and vaginal examinations occur fairly frequently. This is one of the situations in which a close application of anatomical knowledge is necessary, since accurate and intelligent interpretation of vaginal examination findings is one of the midwife's more important responsibilities. A thoughtful and well-planned, though not necessarily long answer to this question may go far to show that the candidate has a real grasp of this essential subject.

Should an anatomical answer be tabulated? There is no real answer to this question, though in fact there is much to be said in favour of tabulation. It saves time and space, it aids clarity of statement and it does not demand a vast and detailed knowledge of correct written English. Though a plan is necessary, the plan is pre-determined. Given neat writing, careful underlining and correct sequences, the total effect is immediately impressive to the reader, i.e., the examiner.

It is possible to write such an answer in essay form, but it is less easy to achieve an effective appearance. English, grammar, paragraphing, punctuation, style in general: all must be impeccable. Even then, some kind of numbered sequence or underlining may appear necessary.

In contrast to Question 1 (page 43), the first part of this answer is set out as an essay.

However the answer is planned, one or two diagrams should be included. Part of Fig. 1(a) (page 27) would be suitable.

**Answer.** *The vagina.* The vagina is a narrow canal extending from the vulva to the uterus. It passes upwards and backwards, being approximately parallel to the pelvic brim. At its lower end it is partially occluded, in the virgin, by the hymen. At its uper end is the cervix uteri, which projects into the vault of the vagina at a right angle. Thus the anterior vaginal wall, which is 7 cm long, is shorter than the posterior wall, which measures 10 cm. The gutter, or recess surrounding the vaginal part of the cervix is, for descriptive purposes, divided into four vaginal fornices. The anterior fornix is shallow, the posterior fornix is deep and the two lateral fornices are intermediate. The anterior and posterior vaginal walls are normally in contact with one another.

The vagina receives its blood supply mainly from the two vaginal arteries, which are branches from the internal iliac arteries. The venous drainage is by a similar route: via the vaginal veins to the internal iliac veins. The lower vagina receives sensory nerves from branches of the pudendal nerves and sympathetic and parasympathetic nerves from the plexus of Lee Frankenhäuser.

The vagina is related anteriorly in its upper half to the base of the bladder and in its lower half to the urethral canal. Posteriorly, adjacent to the uppermost third is the Pouch of Douglas; to the middle third, the rectum; and to the lowermost third, the perineal body.

Above, is the uterus; below, the vagina opens on the vestibule; the parametrium and the ureters lie adjacent to the lateral fornices; below this are the pubo-coccygeus muscles; and, lower again, the transverse perineal and bulbo-cavernosus muscles.

The vaginal walls are made up of an inner layer or lining of squamous epithelium, a vascular layer of connective tissue and two layers of muscle: an inner circular layer and an outer layer of longitudinal fibres. The connective tissue surrounding this carries the blood vessels, lymphatics and nerves of the vagina.

The information to be obtained from a vaginal examination in labour may be summarized as follows:

*In the first stage:*

1. The cervix: its thickness, its consistency, its application to the presenting part and its dilatation.

2. The membranes: their state; if intact, the shape of the bag of forewaters; if ruptured, the colour and quantity of the liquor draining.

3. The presenting part: its identity (usually the vertex); its station, in relation to the ischial spines; other features, e.g., caput succedaneum, moulding, sutures and fontanelles.

The vaginal examination is made for the purpose of determining the features listed above; it is convenient at the same time to note the muscular tone of the vaginal walls, the state of the rectum and certain features of the bony pelvis, namely the character of the sacral curve, the degree of prominence of the ischial spines and the shape and width of the pubic arch.

Finally, the vaginal examination findings must be reviewed in the context of the labour as a whole. The patient's age, parity and history; her progress, her condition and that of the fetus; the uterine contractions and the abdominal examination findings; all these factors must be taken into consideration in order to make a fair assessment from any vaginal examination.

*In the second stage:*

A vaginal examination is not as a rule necessary in a normal second stage, but it should be undertaken if indicated. For the midwife, the commonest indication is failure of the labour to make adequate progress.

The investigations would include ascertaining that the cervix was indeed fully dilated and the membranes ruptured; but the main consideration would be the presenting part, its station and detail of the position, especially if occipito-posterior or occipito-lateral. Caput formation and moulding would also be assessed.

*In the third stage:*

In a case of delay in the third stage (without haemorrhage) it is useful to make a vaginal examination to determine whether or not the major part of the placenta is in the vagina. If it is, digital extraction can be quickly effected; if not, this is the time for a midwife to have the patient seen by a doctor.

This is quite a long answer. It could be shortened by introducing a pattern of tabulation throughout. (Note, however, that tabulation is not the same thing as abbreviation, which is generally not acceptable.) It would be possible also to omit some of the detail: perhaps, detail of the structure of the vagina, or of vaginal examination in the third stage.

This question has been reviewed in some detail, since it is of a type asked fairly often, not only in English, Scottish and Northern Ireland papers, but also in the oral examinations where the conduct of vaginal examinations and the interpretation of their findings provides scope for much useful discussion.

Questions 18 and 19 are very similar indeed to the above; Question 20 is slightly different in its emphasis.

**Q.18. Describe the anatomy of the vagina. What information may be obtained from a vaginal examination in labour?**

**Q.19. What information may be got from a vaginal examination carried out during labour?** *(Scotland)*

**Q.20. Describe the vagina mentioning its anatomical relations. What are the causes of vaginal discharge during pregnancy?** *(Northern Ireland)*

In Q.20 it is clearly necessary to describe as fully as possible the vagina itself, and to write briefly, too, about the related structures. The second part of the question, however, may be covered much more quickly than in the previous questions.

**Q.21. Describe the anatomy of the vagina. Discuss the indications for making a vaginal examination in pregnancy and labour.**

**Q.22. Describe the anatomy of the vagina. Discuss the indications**

**for making a vaginal examination in pregnancy and labour.**
*(Northern Ireland)*

The first part of the answer to these two identical questions so exactly echoes that of the answer to Q.17 that there would be no point in repeating it. The second part is set out below in respect of pregnancy. Vaginal examination in labour, again, is to a great extent covered in the answer to Q.17.

**Answer.** In pregnancy, vaginal examinations are carried out routinely on two occasions: at the first clinic visit and around the 36th week.

At the patient's first visit the obstetrician makes a pelvic examination principally to check that the uterus is enlarged to a size corresponding to the calculated duration of the pregnancy, that it is anteverted and that there are no pelvic tumours.

If the patient has had any recent vaginal bleeding this examination is deferred. While it is unlikely that it would precipitate a miscarriage, if the patient did miscarry, both she and the obstetrician might wonder if there could be a connection.

A second routine vaginal examination is made at about the 36th week, mainly to confirm the adequacy of the pelvis. If the head is engaged, only the lower cavity and outlet need be checked. If not, the obstetrician may make a bimanual examination, noting if the head engages on pressure and investigating the pelvic brim, cavity and outlet.

Sometimes a vaginal examination is indicated at some other stage of pregnancy, e.g., to determine the presentation in case of doubt, or to note ripening of the cervix. As opposed to digital examination per vaginam, the indication for a speculum examination may occur at any stage of pregnancy, typical indications being cervical or vaginal cytology, vaginal discharge and antepartum haemorrhage.

**Q.23. Discuss the indications for vaginal examination in pregnancy and labour.**

This question is included here because, though not strictly

anatomy and physiology, it is so similar to the foregoing one that useful comparisons can be made.

Since the anatomy is not asked, there is now scope for fuller discussion. This could mean either amplifying some of the features discussed above or introducing other, less common indications for vaginal examination.

**Q.24. Describe the cervix uteri and the way in which it opens during the first stage of labour.**

There is a good deal of material to be covered in the first part of this question, and it is thus important to pick out the essentials, and to include only these, as concisely as possible. A list of anatomical headings is an advantage in setting out a concise and orderly answer. Anatomy answers are almost always better with some illustration, and here part of Fig. 1, drawn on a larger scale, would be useful.

**Answer.** *General characteristics.* The cervix uteri, or neck of the uterus, is the lowermost third of the non-pregnant uterus.
*Size.* It is 2·5 cm in length, and the walls are about 1 cm thick.
*Shape.* It is cylindrical, with a spindle-shaped cavity.
*Attitude.* In the anteverted uterus the cervix is directed backwards and downwards.
*Divisions.* The upper half is termed the supravaginal cervix; the lower half, which projects into the vagina, is known as the vaginal portion or portio vaginalis.
*Relations:*
    Anterior: the base of the bladder.
    Posterior: the pouch of Douglas.
    Superior: the corpus or body of the uterus; the cavity of the cervix communicates with the cavity of the body by the internal os.
    Inferior: the vault of the vagina with which the cavity of the cervix communicates by the external os.
    Lateral: the parametrium, the uterine arteries and the ureters.
*Blood supply.* From the two uterine arteries, from the internal iliac arteries. The venous drainage follows the same route.

*Structure:*
(a) Peritoneum. This covers the posterior wall of the supra-vaginal cervix only.
(b) Muscle. A little of the outer longitudinal muscle of the body, but mainly the muscle fibres run circularly. The cervix contains a good deal of fibrous tissue.
(c) Mucosa. The cervix has a lining of mucous membrane, which is continuous at the external os with the skin which lines the vagina. Not uncommonly the mucous membrane extends outside the external os and thus may be seen, per speculum, as a reddened area which readily bleeds. This constitutes a cervical erosion.

In early pregnancy the cervix becomes much more vascular. This leads to an increased secretion from the cervical glands, with, often, a slight mucoid vaginal discharge; and the venous congestion causes the cervix to become softer, and to appear bluish in colour.

In the last few weeks of pregnancy the cervical canal may be partly 'taken up' into the lower uterine segment. This is known as 'ripening' of the cervix.

The same change, occurring during the first stage of labour, is described as effacement or taking up of the cervical canal. In the primigravida, this begins when the contraction and retraction of the uterus, stronger in the upper uterine segment, is sufficient to stretch the lower segment and exert a 'pull' on the region of the internal os. The internal os is gradually dilated, the upper part of the cervical canal is effaced, the membranes separate from the lower segment and a small amount of bleeding occurs from the decidua. This blood, together with the plug of mucus from the cervical canal, is shed. This blood-stained mucus constitutes the 'show' commonly seen at about the onset of labour.

The uterine contractions, shortening the upper uterine segment, exert a pull upon the cervix until the cervical canal is completely effaced. With stronger contractions, the upward pull is now exerted on the external os. If the membranes are ruptured and the cervix closely applied to the fetal head, dilatation is facilitated. The uterine contractions become progressively more frequent, stronger and of longer duration; and this combination of forces effects increasing dilatation of the external os until the cervix is completely dilated and the uterus and vagina form one continuous canal. From the onset of labour this process takes about 12 or 14 hours in a primigravida.

In the multigravida, the process is somewhat quicker, effacement and dilatation occurring at the same time.


**Q.25. Describe the changes that take place in the cervix during pregnancy and normal labour.**

Here the anatomical features of the cervix are not asked. It is necessary, however, to present the physiological changes of pregnancy in somewhat more detail. The first stage of labour might be covered rather more briefly than in Question 24; and, though there may appear to be little to write, the second and third stages of labour must be mentioned.


**Q.26. Describe the umbilical cord. What should a midwife do if the cord prolapses?**

The anatomy of the umbilical cord is short, straightforward and simple enough, except for the candidate who becomes confused over the blood vessels. This difficulty may best be overcome by reviewing the physiology of the cord. The placenta constitutes (among other features) the lungs of the fetus, hence the blood vessels in the cord are comparable to the pulmonary arteries and veins: the umbilical arteries, like the pulmonary arteries, carrying de-oxygenated blood; and the umbilical vein, like its pulmonary counterparts, returning freshly oxygenated blood to the heart. *To* the heart – this is the other clue. All blood vessels carrying blood towards the heart are veins. The umbilical vein, part of the fetal circulation, is carrying blood (oxygenated blood) *towards* the fetal heart, for distribution through the body.

Prolapse of the umbilical cord is one of the major emergencies of midwifery practice. Action comes first: medical aid or flying squad second. Unless the child is known to be dead – but diagnosis is difficult and treatment nil – act as though it were alive.

**Answer.** The umbilical cord is a rope-like structure, extending from the centre of the fetal surface of the placenta to the fetal umbilicus. Though its size may vary considerably, it is normally about 50 cm long and 1·5 to 2 cm in diameter.

The cord contains, normally, three blood vessels. The large vessel is the umbilical vein through which oxygenated blood flows from the placenta to the fetus; the smaller vessels are the two umbilical arteries, which take de-oxygenated blood from the fetus to the placenta. The arteries wind round the vein, giving the cord a twisted appearance. These vessels, together with the vitelline duct, a vestigial remnant of the embryonic yolk sac, are embedded in Wharton's jelly, a jelly-like connective tissue. The cord has a covering of amnion, continuous at the placental end with the amnion covering the placenta and, at the fetal end, with the skin of the child's abdominal wall.

In the event of prolapse of the cord, there are two essential principles in the management of the case.

1. To prevent compression of the cord.
2. To deliver the patient as soon as possible.

The mother is at once placed in Sims' position, she is given Entonox or pure oxygen to inhale, while the foot of the bed is raised on 12-inch blocks. As quickly as possible a message is sent, calling a doctor urgently.

If the patient is in labour, the midwife should introduce two fingers into the vagina, in order to push up the presenting part during contractions. If, in this way, she can maintain good cord pulsation, she must continue this procedure until help arrives.

If there is any cord outside the vulva, it is gently replaced in the vagina, in order to keep it warm; this helps to prevent spasm and consequent constriction of the vessels.

If bed blocks are not immediately available, the patient is placed temporarily in the uncomfortable knee-elbow position.

The patient may be a multigravida, in the second stage of labour. In this case, the midwife should make every effort to hasten delivery: by encouraging the patient to 'push', by herself applying fundal pressure during contractions, or by performing an episiotomy.

This answer needs a diagram in colour. No candidate need hesitate; the drawing is simple, easy and quick; the result surprisingly impressive.

The above account takes into consideration only essentials. It is possible to attempt listening to the fetal heart sounds, but it is not easy; and, whether or not the fetal heart is audible, the management is the same since it is based on an assumption that the fetus is alive. Moreover, the cord pulse provides better evidence whether or not the cord is being compressed.

Compare the next question, Question 27. Here, an anatomical description is not asked; instead, a full account is required, giving the emergency management.

**Q.27. Describe the management of a patient with prolapse of the umbilical cord.** *(Scotland)*

Question 28 reverts to anatomy, but here, the applied anatomy relates only to the neonate, only in emergency and is simply to be 'indicated'.

**Q.28. Describe the anatomy of the umbilical cord and indicate its importance in neonatal emergency treatment.** *(Scotland)*

**Q.29. Describe the structure of the umbilical cord. What complications of the cord may affect the life of the fetus during pregnancy and labour?**

Here the same degree of knowledge and awareness is needed, though the question has a rather more theoretical slant. In the answer set out below the structure of the cord, given in the answer to Q. 26, is not repeated.

**Answer.** The fetus is dependent upon the patency of the umbilical vein, firstly for his oxygen supply and secondly, for less urgent needs such as nutrition. Stretching narrows the lumen of the umbilical vessels; compression may obliterate it completely.

Since the cord vessels are part of the fetal circulation, rupture causes fetal haemorrhage.

These complications may arise in pregnancy and labour.

In the course of external cephalic version, the cord, particularly a rather long cord may become wound round the neck or a limb of the fetus, causing some compression.

A long cord may lie, or, during version, come to lie partially below the presenting part of the fetus. This condition, cord presentation, is potentially highly dangerous since, immediately the membranes rupture, it becomes cord prolapse, which is discussed below.

A short cord is more readily pulled upon, again perhaps during version. This may separate a part of the placenta, causing antepartum haemorrhage, a risk to both mother and fetus.

Very occasionally the fetus, moving freely in the liquor amnii, passes through a loop of cord, thus tying a loose knot. Traction on the cord, whether in pregnancy or labour, tightens this 'true knot', causing severe fetal hypoxia.

Vasa praevia is velamentous insertion of the cord in which the velamentous vessels are lying in the lower uterine segment, below the presenting part of the fetus. Usually the placenta is, in some degree, praevia and antepartum haemorrhage is inevitable. Vasa praevia, being rare, is not usually suspected; but the slightest possibility of fetal distress warrants a Singer's test to determine if there are fetal cells in the blood lost per vaginam. A positive test means that the fetus, as well as the mother, is losing blood. The fetal blood comes from rupture of a velamentous vessel. But even if it does not rupture, a velamentous vessel is easily compressed.

Cord presentation, mentioned above, is not usually diagnosed, though it is occasionally revealed when a chance vaginal examination is made for some other purpose and the cord is palpated in the forewaters. It is generally during early labour that the membranes rupture, converting it into cord prolapse. This is extremely dangerous to the fetus, so it is fortunate that it is generally recognised promptly.

**Q.30. Compare the anatomy of the non-pregnant uterus with that of the uterus at term.** *(Scotland)*

There is no one and only way to answer an anatomy question.

The subject matter is, of necessity, factual and unequivocal; but not its manner of presentation. The answer could be in essay form; and if the essay were clear, interesting and readable the achievement would be admirable and the examiners probably favourably impressed. But most candidates would rather avoid an essay and many would be aware of the temptation to write a meandering and paragraphless rigmarole. Tabulation of some kind is usually easier, shorter and clearer. Tabulation patterns, too, vary; and in this particular answer, where so many features are to be compared, there is much to be said for a complete table. The candidate will think of other subjects which lend themselves to this treatment, e.g., caput succedaneum and cephalhaematoma, placenta praevia and abruptio placentae. (See table on facing page.)

Tables of this kind need ample space; cramping leads inevitably to confusion. Nor is minutely small writing helpful. The calligrapher who transcribed the Lord's Prayer on a sixpence doubtless won his place in the Guinness Book of Records. The candidate who picks up her mapping pen, similarly inclined, will succeed only in exasperating the examiners to whom her script is submitted.

A single page is insufficient. It is much preferable to spread the answer right across two pages, in the manner of a newspaper middle spread. A little extra time will be spent in the planning; but this is more than offset by the time saved in writing, not to mention additional marks gained for the clarity of presentation.

### Q.31. Describe the anatomy of the uterus. What changes does the uterus undergo in pregnancy and labour?

In this question about the uterus, the material required is, in many respects, that set out in the answer to Q.30, but here the emphasis is altered. The list of headings, however, is the same: a useful aide memoire, well worth learning by heart, since it furnishes the outline for so many anatomical answers.

Here are three questions on the anatomy and physiology of the uterine muscle.

| | Non-Pregnant Uterus | Uterus at Term |
|---|---|---|
| General Characteristics | A small hollow muscular organ lying in the centre of the pelvic cavity | A very large muscular organ, filling the pelvic and abdominal cavities and displacing adjacent organs |
| Size | 7·5 cm long, 5 cm wide at widest part and 2·5 cm from front to back | 30 cm long, 22 cm wide and 20 cm deep |
| Weight | 60 g | 900 g |
| Shape | Pear shape, flattened antero-posteriorly | Ovoid |
| Attitude | Anteverted and anteflexed | Upright |
| Divisions | Body = uppermost 4·5 cm, isthmus = 6–7 mm and cervix = lowermost 2·5 cm | Body, now upper segment = about 20 cm, isthmus, now lower segment = about 7 cm; cervix = 2·5 cm |
| Blood Supply | Ovarian arteries to fundus and upper part of body and cervix. Uterine arteries to lower part of body and cervix | All now markedly increased |
| Venous Return | Similar, to ovarian and uterine veins | |
| Nerve Supply | Sympathetic and parasympathetic in Lee-Franken-häuser plexus | |
| Lymph Drainage | Mainly to the internal iliac glands | |
| Structure Peritoneum | An incomplete covering extending anteriorly to the isthmus | Loose attachment to lower uterine segment |
| Muscle | 13 mm thick, firm and hard. Outer longitudinal layer, over fundus. Middle interlacing layer, comprising bulk of muscle. Inner circular layer, around orifices only } Not clearly distinguish-able | 8 mm thick, very soft and vascular. Hypertrophy and hyperplasia of muscle fibres. Muscle layers clearly demarcated |
| Mucous Membrane | Endometrium, varying with phases of menstrual cycle | Decidua, thicker, more vascular and with more glandular activity than premenstrual endometrium |
| Cervix | Firm and hard. Pink in colour. Os closed. | Very soft. Bluish from venous congestion. Os 0·5–1 cm dilated |

**Non-Pregnant Uterus**     **Uterus at Term**

**Q.32. Describe the uterine muscle and its action in all the stages of labour.**

**Q.33. Outline the anatomy of the body of the uterus. Describe the behaviour of its musculature in the three stages of labour.**

**Q.34. Describe the anatomy of the body of the uterus. Describe the muscle action of the uterus in the third stage of labour.**

It is important in all three of these questions to keep a reasonable balance between anatomy and physiology; and at the same time, not to spend too long answering this one question to the detriment of the others in the examination paper. Most candidates know the anatomy of the uterus well, and many might become over-enthusiastic, and write down everything they know about the uterus without stopping to consider whether they could afford the time to do so. Thus it is here, even more than in Question 24, page 58, that thoughtful planning is necessary, with careful selection of material.

**Q.35. Describe the perineal body. How may it be damaged during labour and what can be done to lessen this damage?**

This kind of question has been asked several times in recent years. Now that midwives are expected to use local anaesthesia, perform and sometimes repair episiotomy, it may be predicted, not only that such questions will re-appear in future examinations, but that candidates will be anticipated to have acquired a clearer understanding of the subject.

**Answer.** The perineal body is a wedge-shaped mass of muscular and fibrous tissue and is the point of insertion of most of the muscles of the pelvic floor. It is bounded in front by the lowest third of the posterior vaginal wall and behind, by the anterior part of the anal canal. Its upper part consists of the anterior part of the pubo-coccygeus muscles (pubo-vaginalis). Below this are inserted the two deep transverse perineal muscles. Beneath this again, most of the superficial perineal muscles converge at the central point of the perineum, while, posteriorly is the anterior part of the external anal sphincter.

The blood supply is mainly from the internal pudendal arteries, which are branches from the internal iliac arteries. The nerve supply is by branches from the pudendal nerves.

The perineal body may be damaged during labour in two ways:

1. By over-stretching. This may be:

(a) *prolonged stretching,* as when the second stage of labour, particularly the perineal phase, is prolonged. The same type of excessive stretching occurs when a well-meaning attendant keeps the head on the perineum too long, in an ill-advised attempt to avoid a tear. This unnecessary prolongation can be avoided by a timely and adequate episiotomy.

(b) *repeated stretching,* such as occurs in women of high parity. This is more difficult to avoid, but if the labours are well managed and the patient practises her postnatal exercises conscientiously, her pelvic floor muscles should remain reasonably strong.

(c) *stretching of extreme degree,* as during the birth of an unusually large baby, or one born in the persistent occipito-posterior position. It is to be avoided by episiotomy, with subsequent careful attention to postnatal exercises.

2. By tearing. Severe tearing of the perineal body can occur in precipitate primigravid labour, which is almost impossible to anticipate; in the birth of a large baby, in persistent occipito-posterior delivery, in breech or forceps delivery, in the absence of an episiotomy; and in the case of a patient with a narrow pubic arch. The initial damage is to be avoided by the performing of an adequate episiotomy. Failing this, the prompt and skilled suturing of all perineal tears is valuable. Third degree lacerations should be repaired in an operating theatre.

In the early postnatal period, good perineal care will help to promote healing; again, postnatal exercises, carefully graded, are of value. Finally, all patients, six weeks after delivery, should have the integrity of the pelvic floor fully assessed.

**Q.36. Describe the perineal body. How may this be damaged in labour and what steps can be taken to minimize this damage?**

**Q.37. Describe the perineal body. How may this structure be damaged during labour and what steps may be taken to minimize this damage?**

**Q.38. Describe the perineal body. How may injury to this structure be prevented during the delivery of the infant?**

Note that Questions 36 and 37 are almost identical. Question 38 is very similar, but asks more detail of the management of labour. Again it is important to stress the risk of stretching. Finally, the practical approach to the problem is clearly presented in Question 39 below.

**Q.39. What are the indications for episiotomy? When should a midwife undertake this procedure? Describe the technique employed.**

It has long been the practice in the Central Midwives Boards' examinations to require the candidate to present the practical application of her knowledge of anatomy and physiology. The following question is an admirable example of this approach:

**Q.40. What practical use can be made during pregnancy, labour and following delivery of a knowledge of the fetal skull?** *(Scotland)*

Consideration of such a question incidentally provides an excellent answer to the occasional lament: 'Why do we have to learn so much anatomy?' Every day, in every department of the hospital, time and time again, the midwife is applying her knowledge of anatomy or physiology to some part of her work. Breast feeding, checking antenatal weight gain, examining a placenta, observation of lochia and the giving of analgesic drugs: all these jobs and many more can be carried out intelligently only if the midwife has an understanding of the basic structure or function.

While one candidate says, 'I couldn't possibly write for half an hour on that', another is saying, 'I couldn't possibly cover it in half an hour', and how right she is. This is true of many of the questions set in these examinations. A better, fuller, more detailed, more comprehensive answer could be written in an hour; or two hours or three or four; or, of course, by writing a chapter in a textbook. No: the situation is such that the candidate has 30 or 35 minutes in which to complete *her* answer. Not more than 35 minutes' work is expected of her: thinking, planning, writing and drawing. Where there is a surfeit of subject matter, her selection and discrimination will be important. What she leaves out will, by virtue of *being* left out, count as much as what she puts in.

One fairly short specimen answer to this question is set out below.

**Answer.** Knowledge of the fetal skull is of great value both before and after the child is born.

During pregnancy this knowledge is probably applied most extensively in carrying out routine abdominal examination. The head is by far the most definite and easily recognised part of the fetus, even as early as about the 24th week, when the fetus may first be palpable. The midwife, aware of the shape and size of the head, locates it, and from this foundation she builds up her concept of the fetus as a whole.

First, presentation is identified by the head: in cephalic presentation it is felt over the pelvis; in breech presentation, in the fundus. Later, the degree of flexion is determined. If both poles of the ovoid which is the head are palpable, one higher than the other, the head is flexed; if both poles are at the same level, it is deflexed. Moreover, the presenting diameter of the flexed head actually feels (and is) smaller than that of the deflexed head; and, in due course, the flexed head engages readily, while the deflexed head fails to engage. It is useful, too, to know that this deflexed attitude of the head is the commonest reason for its failing to engage, and that absolute disproportion is relatively rare.

Occasionally, the head cannot be palpated abdominally and the presentation cannot be determined. It may be deeply engaged, when it can be palpated vaginally or rectally, and recognised by its bony hardness.

Spalding's sign of fetal death is dependent upon the knowledge that, while moulding is a factor of labour, here the bones are overlapping as a result of post-mortem changes in the cranial contents.

Because the average normal rate of growth of the fetal skull is known, it is possible to make accurate assessment of the small-for-dates fetus by means of serial ultrasound B-scan.

During labour, feeling the fetal head abdominally gives much the same information as in pregnancy; but now, as the cervix dilates, vaginal examination reveals much more detailed information, all based upon a knowledge of the fetal skull.

Engagement can be determined very accurately by the relationship of the head to the ischial spines. The conformation of the sutures and fontanelles gives exact detail about presentation and position on the one hand and maturity and moulding on the other, e.g., the four sutures meeting at the bregma, and its actual size distinguish it from the posterior fontanelle.

Caput and moulding will reveal useful features about the character of the labour. Knowledge of the structure of the scalp makes fetal scalp blood sampling a practicable procedure, while forceps application, Kiellands rotation and Ventouse extraction involve application of this anatomical knowledge.

**Q.41. Describe the anatomy of the fetal skull. List the abnormalities which may be observed on the first examination of the head of the newborn infant.** *(Northern Ireland)*

Here is a somewhat different approach to this important anatomical subject. As usual, the anatomy is to be applied, even though the abnormalities have merely to be listed. Implicit in the question is the all-important fact that 'fetal skull' by long tradition, means fetal (and, in this instance, neonatal) head. The interpretation 'head' might also be considered in Q.42.

**Q.42. Describe the fetal skull and the changes that occur in it during labour.** *(Northern Ireland)*

# Pregnancy

# Pregnancy

**Q.43. Describe what you consider to be a suitable diet during pregnancy and give reasons for your choice.**

Answers to questions of this type should be clear and definite, and should avoid reference to a 'good' or 'varied' or 'well-balanced' diet. This is nothing to do with pregnancy, and the person who is not pregnant is not to be expected to eat a poor or monotonous or ill-balanced diet.

Unlike the 'how would you advise about diet?' type of question, which must have a simplified and strictly practical answer, this question may be considered from a technical angle, though it should not be too theoretical, and foodstuffs should be considered as well as calories.

**Answer.** Although the 'eating for two' dictum, which implies a piled-up plate, is now out-dated, it is nevertheless true that a pregnant woman should take, in her food, the materials from which not only the child in her uterus will develop, but also the growing uterus itself, and the breasts, and her own blood. But the modification of her diet is rather of quality than of quantity. It should, moreover, be adapted to the changing anatomy and physiology of her body.

While some women may take adequate amounts of essential foods, and need not alter their diet in pregnancy, many do not, and the following points should be emphasized:

1. Extra protein is needed for building all this new tissue. This may take any form the woman pleases, meat, eggs, cheese and milk being the most valuable sources. Fish is good, but usually less concentrated. Peas and beans may be added as supplements to the animal proteins.

2. Extra carbohydrate, in the form of bread, cakes, and biscuits is

not necessary and should be avoided. Obesity, always undesirable, may become a serious hazard in pregnancy. Fresh fruit and vegetables are valuable for their vitamin C content and for their value as 'roughage' since constipation is common in pregnancy. In this respect, bran cereals are of value.

3. Extra fat is not necessary, and indeed is often not well tolerated in pregnancy; fried foods are better avoided.

4. Minerals. Calcium and phosphorus are needed for the development of fetal bones and teeth. Meat, eggs, cheese and particularly milk are good sources. At least one pint of milk should be taken daily.

Iron is needed for both the fetal and maternal haemoglobin, and is found in meat and liver and, in smaller quantities, in dried fruits, spinach and watercress.

Sea-fish is recommended for the iodine it contains.

5. Vitamins. Vitamins A (anti-infective) and D (necessary for the absorption of calcium) are needed, and are available in cod liver oil and similar preparations, or in tablet form, which most women prefer.

6. Water. Most women are more thirsty than usual during pregnancy, and they probably drink rather more, either as water, or in tea and coffee and fruit drinks. In normal pregnancy a woman should be told to drink as much as she wants.

A typical day's menu might be arranged as follows:

Breakfast: Boiled or poached egg
1 slice of toast or crispbread
Tea or coffee

11 a.m.    Coffee with milk

Lunch:     Liver, green vegetables
Stewed fruit
Biscuits and cheese
Tea or coffee

Tea:       Marmite sandwiches, fruit
Tea

Supper:    Soup
Cold meat and salad
Fresh fruit
Tea or coffee

10 p.m.    Horlick's or Ovaltine

**Q.44. What advice would you give on diet in pregnancy?** *(Northern Ireland)*

This is the same question presented from a slightly different angle. The answer should include the same material, with the exception that even the elementary physiology above should be simplified still further and that technical terms would be better avoided. Thus 'body-building' food may be substituted for 'protein'.

**Q.45. What advice would you give to a primigravida during her pregnancy on: (a) the care of the breasts, (b) diet and exercise?**

Compare this question with the two preceding ones. Here the scope is much wider, and whereas in the one case it is possible to spend half an hour considering diet alone, in the other the same subject must be covered in about ten minutes. At the same time the essential points must be included.

In this connection it is a useful exercise to answer a question in full detail, and then to make a précis of the answer, of one-third or one-quarter the length of the original.

**Answer. (a) The care of the breasts**
*Brassière.* The primigravida is advised to wear a brassière which is sufficiently large, which has fairly broad elastic shoulder straps, and which supports the breasts from below without constriction.
*Nipples.* If they are of good shape, no treatment is necessary, except more frequent washing when the breast secretion increases. If they are not very prominent they may be pulled out gently between the thumb and forefinger, once or twice daily. Flat or retracted nipples may be greatly improved by the wearing of Woolwich shells, beginning as early in pregnancy as possible.
*Expression of colostrum.* During the last six weeks of pregnancy the patient may be taught to express gently a little colostrum, twice a day. This clears the ducts, and helps to avoid extreme engorgement at the onset of lactation.

**(b) 1. Diet.** The patient's diet may already contain enough of the foods specially needed during pregnancy, but it would be wise, nevertheless, to advise her as follows:

(a) Extra protein is valuable, the best foods being meat, eggs, fish, cheese, and milk. Peas and beans would be useful in addition.

(b) No extra fat is needed, nor indeed is it well tolerated in many cases. Fried foods are often better avoided.

(c) She should reduce her intake of bread and cakes but should take as much as she likes of fresh fruit and vegetables. 'All-bran' is useful for constipation.

(d) Foods containing calcium, phosphorus and iron should be taken. Meat and eggs and (especially for their calcium content) cheese and milk are good sources.

(e) The foods mentioned in (c) and (d) should provide the necessary vitamins.

(f) As much fluid should be taken as the patient wishes. She will probably be rather more thirsty than usual.

Many pregnant women cannot take a large meal, and small meals, taken more frequently, would be recommended.

**2. Exercise.** Moderate exercise is good, but very strenuous exercise should be avoided. Thus, competitive sports of any description, e.g. tennis, swimming, etc., should be cut out. Walking in the fresh air is good, and so is dancing, again in moderation. Cycling long distances and up hills would be too tiring, but gentle cycling may be preferable to walking or waiting in bus queues with a heavy shopping basket. Similarly, ordinary housework is a good form of exercise, but spring cleaning and moving heavy furniture is too strenuous.

**Q.46. What abnormal constituents of the urine may be found in pregnancy? What may be their significance?**

The routine testing of many specimens of urine, mostly normal, may sometimes seem rather a dreary exercise, even though it is quickly accomplished. That it is, in fact, exceedingly important, is shown by an examination question of this type.

**Answer.** A routine urine test for protein, glucose and ketones is carried out at every antenatal visit.

(a) *Protein.* Protein may be found in the urine specimen examined at the antenatal clinic at any stage of pregnancy.

If the patient has brought up the specimen in a bottle of her own, this may be contaminated with a protein-containing food. Sometimes the bottle is washed scrupulously, but the cap forgotten. In very many clinics, however, the patient brings her urine in a small disposable plastic container which is unlikely to be contaminated and if protein were found in urine in a clean container it could be contaminated by vaginal discharge. This can be ruled out by examining a mid-stream specimen, about which the patient is fully instructed. If the mid-stream specimen is clear there is no further anxiety about the urine, though a vaginal discharge may need investigation and treatment.

The finding of protein in a mid-stream urine signifies one (or both) of two possibilities:

1. Urinary tract infection, when the protein may be present as a constituent of pus. The urine is cloudy and may have an offensive smell. The patient may have symptoms and signs of pyelonephritis, mild or severe. This is common between the 24th and 30th weeks.

2. The protein is plasma protein from the blood: serum albumin and possibly also, serum globulin. The presence of such protein signifies renal damage and is always serious. In early pregnancy this would suggest pre-existing chronic renal disease, which is not very common. In late pregnancy proteinuria would be extremely suggestive of pre-eclampsia which was becoming severe in degree.

3. An uncommon possibility is that this patient suffers from orthostatic proteinuria, a curious condition in which protein is excreted when the patient is up and about, but not when she is at rest. Admission and the examination of an early-morning specimen would give the answer.

(b) *Glucose.* The finding of a trace of glucose is common. It probably indicates a lowering of the renal threshold for glucose, which is common in pregnancy. If it is found more than once, the blood sugar is investigated. This may mean a random or fasting blood sugar estimation or a glucose tolerance test.

The glycosuria may signify a slow assimilation of carbohydrates

– so-called alimentary glycosuria.

The patient may, however, be discovered to be a latent diabetic, in which case diabetes manifests itself in pregnancy but not otherwise, or she may actually be a diabetic. In either case, she must be under expert supervision.

(c) *Ketones.* It is usual but not invariable for the urine to be tested for ketones at every visit. In the few clinics where it is not a routine procedure, the indications are:

  (i)  the patient complains of vomiting
 (ii)  her breath smells of ketones
(iii)  the urine smells of ketones
 (iv)  the specimen contains sugar
  (v)  the patient looks tired and dehydrated
 (vi)  the patient is a diabetic.

The finding of ketones may signify rather worse than usual morning sickness. If vomiting is sufficient to disturb a patient's carbohydrate and fat metabolism, she needs treatment. In severe vomiting there is marked ketonuria and a diminution of urinary chlorides, and the patient is in urgent need of intravenous dextrose saline.

The finding of glucose and ketones together is very suspicious of diabetes.

(d) *Blood.* Haematuria is uncommon in pregnancy. It might occur in severe urinary tract infection in which case the symptoms would be well marked.

(e) *Pus,* in small quantities, is revealed when the finding of protein is being investigated.

(f) *Bile* is found occasionally. Whatever the cause, as, e.g. in hepatitis, the condition is serious.


**Q.47. Describe the examinations that would be carried out on a pregnant woman at 36 weeks.**
**To what points would you pay particular attention at this stage in pregnancy?**

This is a question of a type which might, to the anxious mind of the examination candidate, appear a little ambiguous. Who (she may infer) is meant to be examining this patient? 'To what points would *you* pay attention . . . ?' implies the midwife; but, whatever the midwife's part in antenatal care, the patient is always seen by the doctor at the 36th week.

The candidate should not allow this to disturb her. If – though it is unlikely – there should be any lurking ambiguity in a question and the candidate had made correct and relevant statements and had made her meaning clear, she would certainly not be penalized; on the contrary.

Here, it may reasonably be inferred that doctor and midwife play mutually complementary parts in the examination of this patient; and the candidate might show how this is to be done.

**Answer.** I should first ask the patient how she was feeling and take note of her general condition. She should feel well, enjoy her food, have sufficient sleep at night and take extra rest in the afternoon. Her colour should be good, and she should not appear tired, nor should her face look puffy. I should myself recommend simple treatment for such minor disorders as, e.g. heartburn or constipation. If she complained of headache I should make careful inquiry as to its frequency and severity. It is unlikely to be symptomatic of pre-eclampsia if there are no physical signs present, but it cannot be ignored and the doctor should be informed.

I should estimate her blood pressure and compare it with previous readings. If it has previously been within normal limits it should not now be more than 130/80. If the reading were higher than this, I should re-take it after the patient had had a short rest. If it were still raised I should inform the doctor as the patient may be developing pre-eclampsia, which commonly arises at this stage of pregnancy.

I should test the urine for protein, glucose and ketones. If any one were present I should at once draw the doctor's attention to it. In an uncontaminated specimen the finding of protein at this juncture means either urinary tract infection, or pre-eclampsia reaching a severe degree.

I should weigh the patient and examine her carefully for evidence of oedema. If she had slight swelling of her ankles, worsening by evening and better in the morning, but no other signs of pre-eclampsia, I should not be anxious; I should advise her to try to rest more, with her feet higher than her pelvis, and to avoid standing in queues. If the oedema were more than slight, or if she had oedema of her hands, face or eyelids, or if she had gained 1 kg or more in weight since her last visit two weeks ago, I should tell the doctor, as such oedema is indicative of pre-eclampsia.

Though I should be interested in the abdominal findings, I should probably leave this to the doctor, as he would wish to take his findings into account when carrying out a pelvic examination to assess the adequacy of the pelvis. In a primigravida, the uterus would probably nearly reach the xiphisternum, the vertex would be presenting, the head probably engaged, the fetal back directed anteriorly or laterally, and the fetal heart sounds clear.

Her haemoglobin would have been estimated, and, with labour drawing near, I should be especially interested in this last reading. If it were normal, I should ascertain that the patient had a sufficient supply of iron tablets to last until her next visit; otherwise I should ask the doctor to write a fresh prescription. If the haemoglobin value were low, the doctor would note this. He might prescribe a different type of iron, or additional folic acid.

The doctor would probably examine the patient's heart and lungs at this visit and I should ask him to sign a note of her fitness for inhalational analgesia in labour.

I should notice if the patient seemed calm and placid or anxious and worried, or tired. I should try to make time to have a short chat with her, to give her an opportunity to ask any questions she wished, and to have her feeling secure about impending events, whether she wanted to discuss the onset of labour, breast-feeding, the calling of an ambulance or any other matter.

**Q.48. What particular points should be noted on an antenatal visit at the 36th week of pregnancy?** *(Northern Ireland)*

This question is very similar to the foregoing one, but more straightforward. It should present no difficulty.

**Q.49. A primigravida attends the clinic at the 38th week of gestation. Describe in detail what examinations would be made and what advice should be given to her.**

This question embodies three small differences: this patient is a primigravida; the fetal head should be engaged; and the advice includes checking up on all factors relating to the onset of labour, including arrangements for coming to the hospital.


**Q.50 Discuss the value of antenatal care in making childbirth safe for mother and baby.**

This is the kind of question which could have an answer of almost unlimited length. Moreover, such an answer, unless carefully planned and rigidly disciplined, tends to meander from the point, and may all too easily include such absurdities as the care of the nipples or the treatment of heartburn.

It is a good plan, therefore, to pick out a few really important ways in which regular antenatal care can indeed preserve the life or health of the mother or child, and to concentrate on these points.

**Answer.** So many of the factors endangering childbirth can be discovered and corrected during pregnancy that antenatal care is of immense value in making childbirth safer.

Pre-existing or potential disease is discovered at the earliest possible stage of pregnancy, and, not only is appropriate treatment given throughout the pregnancy, but arrangements are made for the labour and for further treatment afterwards. Thus, asymptomatic bacteriuria is revealed early in pregnancy and, treatment and follow-up being instituted, acute or chronic urinary tract infection may be avoided. Similarly, in cardiac disease, with extra rest the patient begins her labour in the best condition possible, and her cardiac lesion is less likely to become worse; in diabetes mellitus careful management in pregnancy keeps the mother as nearly stabilized as possible, so that complications are less likely and fetal growth better controlled. Arrangements are made for an induced premature labour or a Caesarean section, giving the child a much greater chance of survival. The same principle applies in thyrotoxicosis, tuberculosis and a host of diseases which, unrecognized and untreated, could put mother and child at considerable risk.

Blood examination also brings to light severe anaemias and haemoglobinopathies. The resultant treatment must have saved the lives of many patients who would otherwise have been seriously at risk during labour. Because a routine serological blood test for syphilis is carried out at the first visit the occasional case of undiagnosed syphilis is recognized and treated, the mother's health restored and a healthy child ensured.

Blood grouping enables a compatible transfusion to be given more quickly. Rhesus typing, antibody examination and amniocentesis have made it possible to forecast those cases in which the child may be affected, and to arrange for suitable treatment, while arrangements can be made for any Rhesus negative patient to receive, after labour, an injection of anti-D gamma-globulin to prevent iso-immunization.

The most common serious complication of pregnancy is pre-eclampsia. By estimation of the blood-pressure, urine tests, regular weighing and observation of oedema, this condition is discovered as soon as it arises; with rest, its severity can usually be lessened. The woman who is admitted to hospital with pre-eclampsia usually makes a good recovery herself and may well have a healthy, if small, baby. If she should default from the antenatal clinic, the condition could worsen, eclamptic fits or abruptio placentae might supervene; and not only might the child be stillborn, but the mother herself might die.

The close attention paid to the welfare of the fetus has done much to reduce the perinatal mortality rate. This is true not only of diabetes, pre-eclampsia and blood incompatibilities mentioned above, but also of the small-for-dates fetus, whose progress can be assessed by serial measurement of the bi-parietal diameter by ultrasound B scan and of the urinary oestriol excretion rate.

Patients who attend the clinic regularly and are instructed are ready to report untoward symptoms. Antepartum haemorrhage is one such symptom, and the patient is promptly admitted to hospital. This enables her to have treatment of the best kind if the bleeding worsens, and if, as often happens, it ceases, she is kept at rest and under close observation for as long as is necessary.

Mechanical difficulties with their attendant risks may be foreseen and circumvented. Cephalopelvic disproportion is recognized and carefully assessed, and suitable arrangements are made for the safest type of delivery.

Malpresentations occurring in the latter weeks of pregnancy are noted; in some cases of breech presentation external cephalic version is carried out. This gives the child a much better chance of survival unharmed than breech delivery with its various hazards: and the occasional unstable lie is noted and the patient watched closely, whereas previously both mother and child might have died as a result of obstructed labour.

Finally, the better education of the mother means that she is more likely to report symptoms (which she might otherwise have ignored) and to have earlier and more effective treatment.

### Q.51. How does good antenatal care reduce the perinatal mortality rate?

Antenatal care constitutes one very important aspect of preventive medicine, so it is not surprising to find this question, in many ways similar to the foregoing one, in a Community Health paper.

Perhaps it is a little more difficult to arrive at a satisfactory answer. More care is needed to ensure that only relevant material is included. It is interesting to find, too, a surprising resemblance to Q.50.

The preventive aspect of antenatal care, the routine investigations and their purpose, the ways in which well patients may be kept well; these features of antenatal care occur repeatedly in C.M.B. questions, both in the English and Scottish examinations.

Note the four following examples, all somewhat similar to Q.50 but with varying shifts of emphasis.

### Q.52. What are the aims of antenatal care? Discuss the advantages to be gained by the mother during pregnancy and labour. *(Scotland)*

### Q.53. What are the aims of antenatal care? At what intervals should a healthy pregnant woman be examined?

**Q.54. At what intervals should a pregnant woman be examined? What special observations should be made in the last month of pregnancy, and what advice may be needed?**

**Q.55 Give a list of the common disorders that may be revealed during antenatal care.**
  **What advice would you give to prevent any three of these becoming major disorders?**

**Q.56. At the 36th week a primigravida is found to have a vertex presentation which is not engaged.**
  **Discuss the possible causes and the investigations which should be made.**

In listing the causes of any condition, it is sensible to begin with the common ones and to proceed to those which are relatively rare.

Note that many manoeuvres exist, in all of which the object is to make the fetal head engage by pressure on it in the axis of the pelvic brim. The candidate need describe only the manoeuvre with which she is most familiar.

**Answer.** It is by no means uncommon for a primigravida to be found at the 36th week to have a vertex presentation with the head not engaged. Often the head becomes engaged within the next week. The commonest known cause of non-engagement of the fetal head in a primigravida at about this time is an occipito-posterior or occipito-lateral position of the vertex with poor flexion of the head. The presenting diameter is not the sub-occipito-bregmatic, measuring $9 \cdot 5$ cm, but the occipito-frontal, of $11 \cdot 5$ cm, which enters the 12 cm oblique diameter of the pelvic brim or the 13 cm transverse diameter less easily. In addition, in occipito-posterior position, the bi-parietal diameter of the head lies in the narrow sacro-cotyloid diameter of the pelvis, and this hinders both descent and flexion of the head.

The character of the bony pelvis may hinder engagement. This is noted particularly in West African and West Indian immigrants in whom the ethnic characteristic of a high angle of inclination of the pelvic brim tends to delay engagement, often until after labour is established.

Cephalopelvic disproportion is uncommon, but, if present, will cause the head to remain high. This might occur either with a small or abnormally-shaped pelvis and a child of normal size; or, with a normal pelvis and a very large fetus.

Occasionally, placenta praevia is first suspected when the head fails to engage at the usual time. (Here the head is high because part of the pelvic cavity is occupied by the placenta.) This is unlikely, however, since placenta praevia is much more commonly first manifested by vaginal bleeding at an earlier stage of pregnancy.

Less likely causes of a high head are undiagnosed tumours occupying the pelvic cavity, and, in an unsuspected twin pregnancy, one small head may be deeply engaged, thus preventing the descent of the second.

Sometimes the head fails to engage, and no reason can be discovered.

The procedure of investigation would be as follows:

1. To send the patient to empty her bladder again. This elementary precaution should never be omitted.

2. To inquire as to the patient's bowels. A full rectum or pelvic colon can hinder engagement of the head. If there is any question of constipation an aperient or a suppository should be administered and the patient's abdomen should be re-examined after she has had a bowel action.

3. To examine the patient when she is standing, leaning slightly forwards resting with her hands on the couch.

The attendant should stand behind and slightly to the right of the patient, and should palpate the head. The head may be found to have engaged spontaneously. It may engage easily on downward and backward pressure. In either case there is no disproportion.

It is probable that, at the 36th week, the patient will have a full clinical pelvic assessment. This will reveal to the doctor anything unusual about the pelvis and may show why the head is not engaged.

If the head cannot be made to engage on pressure it is usual for the patient to have an erect lateral X-ray, which will show the antero-posterior diameters of the pelvis and the outline of the fetal head, both equally magnified. The degree of disproportion can thus be assessed and appropriate arrangements made for the labour.

**Q.57. What are the blood examinations which should be undertaken in the care of a pregnant woman?**
**Indicate the significance of these examinations.**

Questions about blood tests undertaken in pregnancy, or about anaemia in pregnant women are asked fairly frequently both in the paper and in the oral examination. Sometimes, as in Questions 58 and 59, it is simply in the form of writing short notes, when it would be appropriate to mention only the tests routinely carried out. Here, however, the whole question is devoted to blood tests and their significance; and, while the regular tests should obviously come first, it would not be incorrect then to mention others.

**Answer.** On the occasion of a patient's first antenatal clinic visit, a specimen of blood is obtained and a number of routine tests are carried out.
1. The haemoglobin value of the blood is ascertained. It should be 12 g or more, allowance being made for the slightly lower values resulting from the hydraemia of pregnancy. Nevertheless, because anaemia in pregnancy is common and, potentially dangerous, this test is of importance. In most clinics this test is repeated at every visit.

Iron deficiency anaemia is common in pregnancy and most obstetricians recommend the routine giving of medicinal iron to all patients. It is still necessary to know at intervals the haemoglobin values, since any anaemic patient who is not responding favourably to iron therapy may have a megaloblastic anaemia resulting from folic acid deficiency.
2. The patient's ABO blood group is determined and the Rhesus type is ascertained. This knowledge is useful since, if the patient should suffer an ante- or post-partum haemorrhage, blood of the

correct type may, without delay, be obtained for cross-matching.

3. A serological test is carried out to exclude, or, occasionally, to diagnose syphilis. If syphilis is confirmed, the patient is at once given treatment. This not only cures the condition, but ensures that the child will not be affected.

4. If the patient's blood is Rhesus negative, it is examined for antibodies, which might affect the fetus adversely. If no antibodies are present, monthly tests are repeated from about the 26th week. In most cases antibodies are not present and, after delivery, the patient can be given anti-D gamma-globulin to guard against Rhesus iso-immunization.

If the patient already has antibodies, treatment can be arranged in an attempt to safeguard the child.

5. If the patient is a West African or a West Indian immigrant, her haemoglobin will be examined to see if it is of the normal adult type, or if any of the red cells show a sickling characteristic. A sickle 'trait' is not necessarily serious, but it is helpful to know its existence, since it may be transmitted to the child. Occasionally a patient is found to have sickle cell disease, in which case her pregnancy is very hazardous.

When a patient has glycosuria on more than one occasion, she may have either a fasting or a random blood sugar estimation, or a glucose tolerance test. If she is found to be a diabetic, she will need specialized care during pregnancy.

**Q.58. Write** *short* **notes on** *four* **of the following:**
(a) **Auscultation of the fetal heart**
(b) **Blood tests in pregnancy**
(c) **Engagement of the fetal head**
(d) **Episiotomy**
(e) **Oedema in pregnancy**
(f) **Care of the umbilical cord**

**Q.59. Write** *short* **notes on** *four* **of the following:**
(a) **Accidental haemorrhage**
(b) **Rubella in pregnancy**
(c) **Postpartum haemorrhage**

**(d) Third degree tear of the perineum**
**(e) Blood tests in pregnancy**
**(f) Prodromal (warning) symptoms of eclampsia**

See also chapter on Short Questions, page 172.

**Q.60. Describe what examination you would make of the breasts of a pregnant woman in order to assess her ability to feed her baby at the breast.**

**How can simple treatment during pregnancy prevent some of the early troubles of lactation?**

This is one of a great variety of questions about the breasts and lactation. It is practical in nature and should present no difficulty.

**Answer.** To assess a woman's ability to breast-feed her baby, a careful examination of the breasts is necessary.

Well-marked pregnancy changes – vascularity, pigmentation and secretion would be in favour of adequate breast activity later.

The deep pigmentation seen in the nipples and areolae in some brunettes is also favourable, as the nipples are usually tougher and less likely to become tender or sore; whereas in some white-skinned red-haired women there is very little pigmentation and the nipples are accordingly more sensitive.

The shape and size of the nipple are of considerable importance in assessing the likelihood of successful breast-feeding. Sometimes the nipple is so small that it would be difficult for the child to grasp, and occasionally it is very large, presenting the same difficulty, especially to a small baby. A nipple of medium size is obviously preferable.

The nipple should also be well protracted. It may appear reasonably prominent but retract on compression of the areola, and this would make feeding difficult. It may, on the other hand appear rather flat at first, but become prominent as a result of handling. This is much more satisfactory.

The skin of the breasts is examined carefully. The more elastic the skin the less likely is the onset of lactation to be accompanied by severe engorgement and tension.

The physical signs in favour of successful lactation then would be well-marked pigmentation, a nipple of medium size, well protracted, and an elastic skin. In such patients special treatment of the breasts during pregnancy is unnecessary.

In assessing a patient's ability to breast-feed her baby, in addition to this physical examination, it is necessary to ascertain the patient's own wishes in the matter. However excellent her physical make-up, she will feed her baby successfully only if she has a genuine desire to do so.

In the care of the breasts during pregnancy all patients are recommended two simple measures:
1. To wear a brassière which is large enough and which supports the breasts from beneath, without constriction. Moderately wide elastic shoulder straps are usually found to be comfortable.
2. Apart from ordinary washing, to make certain in the latter weeks of pregnancy that the sticky secretion is washed off with soap and hot water, once or twice daily. Otherwise a crust forms, which may make the nipple a little sore.

In addition some authorities recommend that all patients should be taught to express a little colostrum from the breasts, twice daily, during the last 6 weeks of pregnancy. This clears the ducts and, later, allows the milk to flow more easily, thus avoiding in turn extreme tension, back pressure within the alveoli, and, ultimately, failure of lactation.

Flat or retracted nipples may be greatly improved by the regular wearing of Woolwich shells carefully fitted over the nipples, inside the brassière. The shells are worn for gradually increasing periods and are soon quite comfortable if worn all day. The earlier in pregnancy the patient begins to wear them, the better will be the chance of improving her nipples.

Nipples which are only slightly retracted may be improved by manipulation. They are pulled out and rolled gently between the thumb and forefinger, and the patient should persevere with this gentle manipulation twice daily, again over as long a period as possible.

If the nipples are of good shape and severe engorgement can be avoided, lactation may well be established without any trouble.

**Q.61. Describe the anatomy of the breasts. How is lactation initiated?**

**Describe the help you would give to a primipara who wishes to breast feed.**

We are at present witnessing a great renewal of interest in breast feeding. Many more patients are anxious to breast feed successfully.

At the same time it is reasonable to anticipate more examination questions on the subject.

At a first glance, Q.61 may appear to demand a long and detailed answer; but this is not necessarily the case. First, the answer, as so often happens, represents a total of half an hour's work: second, the help is to be given to a primipara: not a primigravida; it is reasonable to suppose that the baby is born and that postnatal but not antenatal help is needed.

**Q.62. How may twin pregnancy be diagnosed? What complications may arise in twin pregnancy and labour?**

This is, on the whole, a straightforward question, but, in answering the first part, the candidate should try to discriminate between valuable evidence and possible misleading factors.

Although it might at first seem appropriate to present the very early mode of diagnosis first further consideration would veto this. This is a midwifery examination and the candidate would do better to begin with her own observations and set out what is in fact the most usual way for a twin pregnancy to come to light. This point applies even more strongly in the somewhat similar Q.66 below, in which *only* the midwife's observations are needed.

**Answer.** The first clinical feature that would give rise to a suspicion of twin pregnancy would probably be a uterus larger than normal for the supposed stage of pregnancy. The suspicion would be rather stronger if the patient had a family history of twins.

The midwife should, however, first check the patient's dates. The date of the first day of the last normal menstrual period should be reviewed, together with the duration of the menstrual cycle and, if known, the date of 'quickening'. If the gestation period appears correct and the uterus is indeed unduly large, the patient being of ordinary build, the two main possibilities are multiple pregnancy and hydramnios.

The large uterus might be noted as early as the 22nd to 24th week. Not for another month or six weeks would the midwife be likely to palpate two fetuses.

By the 28th to 30th week, the midwife's suspicions might be stronger. On abdominal inspection, the uterus would still be unduly large and, perhaps, rounded in shape and unusually prominent.

On palpation, there are two important signs:
1. If two hard, round, fetal heads can be felt with certainty, the patient clearly has more than one fetus in the uterus.
2. Three 'poles' may be felt; whether they are recognizable as two heads and one breech or two breeches and one head is immaterial.

Feeling a multiplicity of fetal parts is suspicious, as is the feeling of a small head (in this large uterus). Neither is diagnostic.

*Auscultation.* The fetal heart sounds are liable to be most misleading. One fetal heart may be audible over a surprisingly wide area; twin fetuses may have hearts beating at about the same rate. The best auscultatory evidence is hearing fetal heart sounds in two widely separated areas, with a silent zone intervening.

If twin pregnancy is suspected on any of these clinical findings, either an X-ray or an ultrasound scan will confirm the diagnosis.

A much earlier diagnosis might be made on ultrasound scan:
1. If, in early pregnancy, the uterus were noted to be too large, or to be growing too rapidly.
2. If a patient having a marked family history of twins requested an early diagnosis.
3. By chance, in a scan conducted for some other purpose.

## Complications of pregnancy

Minor complications are common. Heartburn and digestive disturbances are often aggravated. Pressure symptoms will probably be worsened, particularly ankle oedema and varicosities. The patient often feels large and cumbersome, she may have distressing backache and the additional weight she carries is tiring; often she is dyspnoeic.

Other complications are more serious. Labour tends to be premature. If it begins at the 36th or 37th week, the babies, though small, will have a good chance of survival. Sometimes, however, labour begins at the 30th or 32nd week, when their chances are much poorer.

Pre-eclampsia is commoner than in single pregnancy; severe or even fulminating pre-eclampsia may develop soon after the 30th week, greatly increasing the hazards to mother and fetuses.

Severe anaemia is a further risk to be guarded against, since the two fetuses make a much greater demand on the mother's supply of iron.

In monozygotic twin pregnancy, one fetal sac may become polyhydramniotic. This not only aggravates the pressure symptoms, adding further to the mother's discomfort, but increases the risk of premature labour.

### Complications of labour

In the first stage:

Though usually short, the first stage may be prolonged with poor uterine contractions, the membranes may rupture early, with the escape of much liquor, and particularly if the labour is premature, prolapse of the cord is possible.

In the second stage:

Transverse or oblique lie of the second child.

Undue delay between the two births, with hypoxia of the second child.

Prolapse of the second cord.

Rarely, some placental separation, with intrapartum haemorrhage.

Very occasionally, expulsion of the placenta between the two births, when the second child may be stillborn.

Very rarely indeed, twin locking.

In the third stage:

The placental site is very large and, if uterine contractions are not good, there is a risk of massive postpartum haemorrhage.

**Q.63. How can multiple pregnancy be diagnosed?**
**What antenatal complications could occur?** *(Northern Ireland)*

A very similar question, the difference being that the complications are restricted to the antenatal period.

**Q.64. What complications may occur in a twin pregnancy during the antenatal period? How may these complications be prevented?**

In Question 64, much of the same material is covered. Here, however, since the diagnosis is not required, the complications, and their prevention, i.e., the special management of twin pregnancy should be considered more fully. As in the two preceding questions, care is needed to include only relevant material.

**Q.65. Describe the investigation of a patient with excessive abdominal enlargement at the 30th week of pregnancy.** *(Scotland)*

This question on the other hand, deals entirely with diagnosis, which, including the differential diagnosis from polyhydramnios needs to be explained in detail.

Here are two more questions dealing with multiple pregnancy and labour.

**Q.66. What would make you suspect a multiple pregnancy?**
**Discuss the antenatal complications and the management of a twin pregnancy.**

In the first part, the emphasis is on the midwife's ability to make a provisional diagnosis. The presentation would require the clinical material in the answer to Q.62, perhaps slightly elaborated, and omitting, of course, the part dealing with radiography and sonar.

Is there any possible ambiguity lurking in the second part of the question? Could 'the management of a twin pregnancy' conceiv-

ably mean 'the management of twin pregnancy and labour' ? The
possibility is remote. It is true that in the past we have had chapter
headings in books and lecture subjects in lists, entitled 'Twin
Pregnancy' and covering labour as well; and, indeed, examination
questions with this wording and meaning.

Here the candidate need feel no anxiety.

1. It is not 'twin pregnancy' in the abstract, but '*a* twin pregnancy'; a particular one. The inclusion of the indefinite article
creates a subtle change of emphasis, indefinable but unmistak-
able.

2. The candidate may use her common sense: the answer is quite
long enough without including the management of labour.

3. Question papers are set by panels of experts: experts at their
own subject and widely experienced in knowing how to word a
question in order to elicit a particular answer. For the most part
their phrasing is impeccable; very exceptionally, an ambiguous
question is overlooked. After all, none of us is perfect. But, if an
ambiguous question *is* set, it is not the candidate's fault; and she
will never be penalized. If she has answered a fair interpretation of
the question, her answer will be fairly marked.

Finally, from Scotland comes a question of absolute clarity on
this same subject:

**Q.67. Describe the management of labour in a patient with a twin
pregnancy.** *(Scotland)*

# Labour

# Labour

**Q.68. When should a midwife make a vaginal examination during labour? What information could she obtain?**

The first part of the question – the indications for a vaginal examination in labour – requires careful thought.

The fact that in many maternity hospitals every patient has two or more vaginal examinations during her labour may give the impression that these examinations are an essential part of the conduct of any labour. In fact the majority of these vaginal examinations are made for teaching purposes, and, as such, they are a necessary part of the training of the student midwife; and, in addition, they often provide the young staff midwife with valuable experience: but they do not necessarily benefit the patient.

On the other hand, there are many occasions when a vaginal examination is the only means of ascertaining facts which the midwife must know in order to conduct the labour efficiently. In planning an answer to this question, all these points should be taken into account.

The second part of the question is straightforward. The findings are best recorded in the order in which the structures in question are palpated, and these findings may conveniently be tabulated. A clear diagram is an advantage, though not an essential. Question 17 in the Anatomy and Physiology section is very similar to the latter part of this question.

**Answer.** The indication for a vaginal examination is that certain information is necessary for the proper conduct of the labour, and that such information cannot be obtained by any other means. Normal labours may occasionally be conducted without any vaginal examinations, and in some cases a vaginal examination is indicated only to detect a suspected abnormality.

The midwife would need to make a vaginal examination on the following occasions:

### A. In normal labour

1. In the occasional domiciliary case, if the midwife proposed to leave the patient for a while, she would first ascertain the degree of dilatation of the cervix.

2. It is wise also to ascertain the dilatation of the cervix before giving an enema to a multipara who is in established labour.

3. If pethidine is to be administered to relieve pain and spasm, it is better not to give it near the end of the first stage and by vaginal and other examinations the labour can be fully assessed.

4. A patient who is 'bearing down' is usually in the second stage, but sometimes, in a mistaken anxiety to make good progress a woman will 'push' before the first stage is completed. A vaginal examination will serve a double purpose here. Not only can the midwife discover whether or not the cervix is fully dilated; but in some cases she can also slip the anterior lip of the cervix over the advancing head, and so prevent it from becoming bruised and oedematous.

5. During epidural analgesia, the patient does not feel the transition from first to second stage in the same way, and thus cannot help the midwife. As epidural analgesia becomes more popular, however, midwives are gradually learning to appreciate that the second stage is in progress, though less obviously. Sometimes a vaginal examination is necessary, to be sure about this.

6. Twin labours are usually conducted by a doctor, but a midwife may find that she is the senior person present. In such circumstances the midwife, having ascertained by abdominal examination that the second child is lying longitudinally, should make a vaginal examination and rupture the second bag of membranes to hasten the birth.

### B. To discover or confirm a suspected abnormality.

1. In any labour where the presenting part does not fit well, either in the uterus, or in the pelvis, the umbilical cord may prolapse when the membranes rupture. Thus in breech presentation, or in

an occipito-posterior position with a high, deflexed head, a vaginal examination should always be made when the membranes rupture.

2. To ascertain the presentation where there is doubt. It is sometimes very difficult to distinguish abdominally, e.g. a breech with extended legs, with the breech engaged, from a vertex presentation, with the head deeply engaged.

3. In a case of prolapse of the cord it is necessary to assess the dilatation of the cervix; or it may be necessary to push up the presenting part per vaginam, in order to avoid compression of the cord.

4. If the second stage of labour is prolonged, vaginal examination is necessary to discover any mechanical factor which may be responsible for the delay. The head may be discovered in a persistent occipito-posterior position, or deep transverse arrest may be diagnosed.

5. Although it is not common teaching, a vaginal examination may be of value during the third stage of labour, if it is difficult to recognize abdominally whether or not the placenta is in the vagina.

The information to be obtained from a vaginal examination may be tabulated thus:

(a) The vaginal walls: their muscle tone.

(b) The cervix: its thickness, or thinness; the degree of dilatation; its elasticity; and its application to the presenting part.

(c) The membranes: their state; if intact the shape of the bag of forewaters; if ruptured the amount and colour of the liquor draining.

(d) The presenting part: identification; its station, in relation to the ischial spines; special features, e.g. sutures: fontanelles: caput succedaneum: moulding.

(e) The pelvic cavity and outlet: the convergence of the lateral pelvic walls; the prominence of the ischial spines; the width of the pubic arch; and possibly the mobility of the coccyx.

Whenever a vaginal examination is to be made, as much information as possible should be discovered, and the vaginal findings should be recorded and assessed carefully, taking into consideration the preceding abdominal examination findings, the character of the uterine contractions and the labour as a whole.

### Q.69. Describe the management of twin labour. What complications may occur?

In answering a question such as this it is quite impossible to mention every point in the conduct of the entire labour. It is wise, therefore, to cut to a minimum any material which relates to the management of *any* labour (e.g. aseptic and antiseptic technique) and to concentrate on the particular points relating specially to a twin labour.

**Answer.** Most commonly both fetuses present by the vertex at the onset of twin labour, and this variety will be considered.

#### The management of the first stage
This differs little from that of any normal labour. The careful differentiation of the two fetal hearts may take a little longer. It has been suggested that over-distension of the uterus may lead to uterine inertia, but this is not the case in the majority of twin labours, in which the uterine contractions are good. If it is not the case, a long labour may be anticipated, and the usual procedures in the management of such a labour (e.g. the correction of ketosis, the administration of extra sedatives or analgesics) would be adopted.

When the membranes rupture, at whatever stage, it is wise to make a vaginal examination immediately, as there is a greater likelihood of prolapse of the cord with a small presenting part.

Preparation should be made for the reception and resuscitation of two babies, who may be either preterm or small-for-dates or both.

#### The second stage
This is conducted as in any labour until the first child is born, when (as soon as respiration is established) it is wise to ascertain that the ligature or clamp on the maternal end of the cord is firm. It would be possible (though unusual) for a second of monozygotic twins to bleed by this route, and this small precaution will avoid such a risk. Identity labels, stating that this is the first twin, should be fastened round the child's wrist and on the maternal end of the cord. The

child is put in a warm cot.

The most essential single item in the management of this labour is to examine the mother's abdomen immediately, to ascertain that the second fetus is lying longitudinally. There is a definite risk that an oblique lie may develop during this stage of the labour and it must be corrected as quickly as possible in order to avoid the grave complication of obstructed labour. Usually a doctor is present, but not always. The midwife would proceed in the same way. If she discovers an oblique lie, she should immediately correct it – it is not, as a rule, difficult to do so – and rupture the membranes in order to maintain the longitudinal lie.

If the lie is longitudinal the fetal heart sounds are counted, and the patient is left to rest for a few minutes. Usually the contractions soon begin again, and the second child is born within a short time. The midwife would probably give an intravenous injection of $0 \cdot 5$ mg ergometrine at the birth of the anterior shoulder of the second child. It is likely there will be an X-ray, showing that this is not a case of triplets, but, if there were doubt the ergometrine would be withheld. The birth should be carefully controlled, since too rapid passage through the already dilated birth canal may result in intracranial haemorrhage.

If the second child is not born within about fifteen minutes of the first, the lie being longitudinal, delivery should be hastened by artificial rupture of the membranes. Otherwise there is a risk that the cervix may reform and the labour would then be much delayed with a second 'first stage'.

The second infant and cord should have similar identification labels.

### The third stage
This is conducted in the usual way, but there is an increased risk of postpartum haemorrhage. If the uterine retraction should be inadequate, haemorrhage would be very severe on account of the large placental site. It is for this reason that a powerful oxytocic drug is given as early as possible.

Finally, if the babies are of the same sex, a close examination of the placenta is necessary to ascertain whether the twins are monozygotic or dizygotic.

**Q.70. What are the causes and signs of fetal distress in labour?**

This question may, at a first glance, appear to require only a very short answer.

However, in the first place, there are many ways in which fetal distress may occur, and it is a good plan to give a brief explanation of this in each of the cases mentioned.

Furthermore, the signs of fetal hypoxia, as it is usually termed, are of considerable practical importance. This is a field in which the midwife may easily have more scope for intelligent observation than the doctor. It is she who remains with the patient during the greater part of the labour, and it is she who thus has the best opportunity to appreciate normal fetal heart sounds and any early deviation from the normal pattern. This is a considerable responsibility and the midwife should be prepared to discuss and evaluate clinical signs of fetal hypoxia.

**Answer.** Fetal distress occurs when the oxygen supply to the fetus in utero is diminished to a dangerous degree.

Before reaching the fetal circulation the oxygen must pass via the maternal lungs and blood stream to the placental site and then in the fetal blood through the capillaries of the chorionic villi, the placental veins and the umbilical vein. Many factors, especially in labour, may interfere with the transmission of oxygen, and these causes of fetal hypoxia may be classified as follows:

1. *In the mother:* severe cardiac or pulmonary disease or anaemia with poor oxygenation of the blood: eclamptic fits, during which deep cyanosis occurs.

2. *At the placental site.* Very strong and frequent uterine contractions, especially when the uterus does not relax sufficiently between contractions.

3. *In the placenta.* Partial separation, particularly in abruptio placentae. Gross infarction, as in severe pre-eclampsia. Marked calcification, as may be present in a postmature labour. Compression of the placenta following rupture of the membranes and loss of liquor amnii.

4. *In the cord.* Compression of the umbilical cord may occur in the prolapse of the cord, and also during breech delivery.

5. Fetal distress may also result from intracranial birth trauma, or

occasionally from the administration to the mother of drugs which depress the vital centres.

The signs of fetal hypoxia:

1. Alterations in the fetal heart sounds are in many instances the most valuable evidence.

(a) the heart rate slows, and does not return to normal between contractions. A fall of 20 beats per minute below the previous rate is serious.

(b) sometimes a transient rise in the fetal heart rate is noted. A rise of 20 beats per minute would give rise to anxiety.

(c) the rate, or rhythm, or both may become irregular. This is very serious.

(d) the sounds become fainter, and if the condition cannot be relieved quickly, the heart sounds soon cannot be heard.

2. Meconium staining of the liquor amnii or the passage of meconium per vaginam is, in some cases, significant of fetal distress. In a breech delivery it was at one time considered to signify only the inevitable compression of the abdomen and buttocks but it is now appreciated that the passage of meconium in breech labour may be of serious import. The passage of meconium-stained liquor when the fetal heart sounds are strong and regular suggests that there has been a transient occasion of fetal distress sometime earlier.

3. In a fetus already distressed it is sometimes noted that the fetal movements become excessive ('tumultuous') shortly before they cease.

4. With modern monitoring equipment, it is possible to judge more exactly the condition of the fetus.

Continuous monitoring of the fetal heart will reveal much more of the small variations in rate and rhythm than is possible by intermittent listening through a monaural stethoscope. Thus a tracing which shows slowing during a contraction with a quick return to normal rate (Type 1 dip) is not abnormal. Slowing of the heart with a short delay before rising to a normal rate (Type 2 dip) is characteristic of early fetal hypoxia.

5. The taking of a small quantity of fetal scalp blood and the estimation of its pH value will show, within very narrow margins, whether or not delivery is urgently necessary. A pH of 7·25 or

more is considered satisfactory, if a little low; pH values between 7·20 and 7·25 indicate that the fetus is in danger so delivery is necessary; while a reading of less than 7·20 is an urgent indication for immediate delivery.

**Q.71. What are the signs of fetal distress? How should a baby born in a state of severe asphyxia be treated?**

**Q.72. How would you diagnose fetal distress during labour? How should a baby born in a state of severe asphyxia be treated in the first 24 hours of its life?**

These two questions are similar, but of a rather more practical nature. They serve to remind the candidate to think carefully about the child when similar conditions may obtain immediately before and immediately after birth.

**Q.73. How is occipito-posterior position diagnosed during pregnancy and labour?**
**Describe the management of this condition during labour.**

This is one example of the kind of 'borderline' condition which might well be the midwife's responsibility, but which could easily overstep the boundary of normality and require the help of the obstetrician. Now that practically all women have a hospital delivery the distinction is, in some respects, less important, though the midwife's basic responsibilities remain.

In the first part of this answer it should be borne in mind that there will be two sets of findings; those where the head is flexed and those where such flexion is incomplete. A clear distinction between the two should be made both in the abdominal examination findings and, in respect of labour, in those found on vaginal examination.

The second part of the question brings out the matter of responsibility mentioned above, in this instance serving to show the complementary functions of doctor and midwife. It is the midwife who has the patient under continuous observation and she is usually able to decide whether progress is normal or not. It follows that in order to consult a doctor in reasonable time she should know the abnormalities which may arise, and be able to detect them early.

**Answer.** An occipito-posterior position is usually diagnosed, whether during pregnancy or labour, by abdominal examination. A doubtful diagnosis may be confirmed during labour by vaginal examination.

*Abdominal examination.* Inspection of the abdomen reveals a uterus which is ovoid longitudinally, but often with some prominence in the region of the fundus and flattening around the umbilicus. Fetal movements may be clearly visible.

Palpation would reveal either:

(a) the head is flexed and, in late pregnancy and in labour, probably engaged. The sinciput is felt as a distinct prominence on one side above the pubic bone; or,

(b) the head is not well flexed: in this case it is probably not engaged. If the occiput is markedly posterior the narrow bitemporal diameter of the head is felt; if the occiput is more laterally placed, the deflexed head feels wide with occiput and sinciput at the same level.

In all cases fetal limbs are felt on both sides of the abdomen, and the resistance of the child's back is either felt with difficulty, in one or other flank; or is not felt at all.

Auscultation: the fetal heart sounds can be heard at and near the mid-line below the umbilicus; and also in one or other flank. In cases where the fetal back cannot be recognised, the hearing of the fetal heart sounds in one flank is a useful indication that the back is directed to that side.

During labour it would be suspicious if the membranes ruptured early: if the fetal head remained high; if the contractions were poor and progress slow, particularly if the mother were suffering severe backache, which is almost diagnostic.

All this might be readily confirmed by abdominal examination, as described above, but sometimes the determining of the fetal position by this means might be inconclusive.

In this case, a vaginal examination is necessary for confirmation.

(a) with good flexion, the membranes are more likely to remain intact longer; the head is felt at the level of the ischial spines with the sagittal suture in one or other oblique diameter; the posterior fontanelle may be just felt posteriorly with very good flexion; the anterior fontanelle is probably palpable anteriorly;

(b) if flexion is not good the membranes may well have ruptured early: the head is above the spines and the anterior fontanelle will be palpated centrally. The posterior fontanelle will not be felt. As labour advances a large caput may be felt.

*The management of labour*

In some cases, an occipito-posterior position does not appear to affect the course of labour adversely. The contractions are good, the fetal head descends and easily makes a long rotation in the second stage and, at the end of labour, mother and child are perfectly well. In a case of this kind, the management of labour does not differ from that in an occipito-anterior or occipito-lateral labour. In the late first stage and second stage, abdominal examination will reveal the increasingly anteriorly directed fetal back and during delivery, restitution and the birth of the shoulders may be anticipated accordingly.

Often, however, this malposition causes the labour to be more painful and the patient suffers very severe backache. This is most effectively relieved by epidural analgesia, which the anaesthetist will induce as soon as this characteristic back pain becomes evident.

If labour is progressing slowly an intravenous dextrose infusion is set up in order to avoid ketosis, which is unpleasant and undesirable for the mother and which puts the fetus at risk of hypoxia.

If the fetal head remains high and deflexed, a vaginal examination should be performed immediately the membranes rupture to determine whether or not the cord has prolapsed.

The uterine contractions, maternal pulse and fetal heart sounds should be monitored frequently, while close observation is made of flexion and descent of the fetal head. The labour may need to be terminated by Caesarean section for fetal distress, prolapse of cord, or extension of the head into a brow presentation.

Occipito-posterior position is a common cause of delay in the second stage, the head being arrested with the occiput lateral (deep transverse arrest), obliquely posterior or persistently posterior. The usual treatment is a Kiellands forceps rotation and delivery, though sometimes the Ventouse vacuum extractor is used. For spontaneous persistent occipito-posterior delivery a deep episiotomy is needed.

The child should be observed in a special care unit for evidence of intracranial birth trauma.

**Q.74. What are the possible courses of labour in a primigravida with the fetal head in the occipito-posterior position?**
**Describe your management of such a case.**

The abnormal features of occipito-posterior labour receive so much emphasis that it is not surprising that the possibility of normal progress should sometimes be overlooked. Furthermore, some cases must go unrecorded, since many patients do not come into hospital until labour is well established; and by this time the fetal head may have rotated to an occipito-lateral position.

In answering this question, it is well to consider these normal cases first. Then the complicating factors may be set out.

The latter part of the question differs from that of Q.73 in one respect: 'your' management as opposed to 'the' management. Thus, the midwife's management is to be set out in some detail; the complications requiring medical help must obviously be mentioned; while the nature of the doctor's work need only be briefly outlined.

**Q.75. How would you diagnose an occipito-posterior position during labour? Describe the midwife's care of a young primigravida with an occipito-posterior position during the first stage of labour.**

**Q.76. Outline briefly the complications which can occur in a case of occipito-posterior position during labour.**

These two questions give additional emphasis to the points mentioned above: that, while occipito-posterior labour can well be normal, many complications, dangerous to mother and child, may arise. It lays a heavy responsibility upon the midwife, it demands of her a high degree of intelligent anticipation and it is hardly surprising that it should remain an appropriate examination subject.

**Q.77. What are the causes of delay in the second stage of labour in a woman who has previously had a normal labour?**

It may seem that there is not much to be said in answer to this question. If, however, it is to constitute half an hour's work – thinking, planning and writing, the subject clearly merits careful consideration.

The factors which might be responsible for the delay should be arranged in order of frequency, and in each case a few words of explanation should be added.

It is necessary, too, to distinguish between delay and obstruction, where delivery is mechanically impossible. Moreover, the causes of obstructed labour, e.g. brow or shoulder presentation, gross disproportion, would be recognized before the second stage had begun, and would therefore not be relevant in any case.

**Answer.** The second stage of labour is probably unduly prolonged if, after half an hour, a multigravid woman is not delivered. This may be due to any of the following causes:

1. Occipito-posterior position of the vertex. This is the commonest cause of prolongation of the second stage in these circumstances; it should always be suspected when delay occurs in a woman who has previously had a normal labour.

The fetal head is probably deflexed, so that a larger longitudinal diameter is presenting. It may be in any one of three positions:

(a) persistent occipito-posterior, when the sinciput has been the first part to meet the resistance of the pelvic floor, and has thus been rotated forwards to the symphysis, the occiput being carried to the hollow of the sacrum.

(b) unreduced occipito-posterior position, when no rotation has occurred and the fetal head is arrested with the occiput obliquely posterior.

(c) the head may have attempted unsuccessfully a long (⅜ circle) rotation, and have become arrested with its long diameter transverse. This is especially liable to develop if the ischial spines are at all prominent. If this patient had, at her previous confinement, had an occipito-anterior position, the problem would not have arisen.

2. Poor uterine contractions. In almost all cases of delay in the second stage, the uterine contractions are weaker and/or less frequent than normal. If the contractions had been better, progress, even with an occipito-posterior position, might have been normal.

3. A malpresentation, such as a breech or face presentation might prolong the second stage though again only if the uterine contractions are poor. With good contractions progress might well be normal.

4. Slight disproportion, especially at the pelvic outlet. This is uncommon, but it could prolong the second stage of labour in a multigravida who had a larger child than before.

5. A short umbilical cord. A relatively or absolutely short cord is a somewhat rare cause of delay in the second stage of labour.

In the majority of these cases, if the uterine contractions were strong there would be no delay.

**Q.78. What are the common causes of delay in the second stage of labour?**
**How may they be recognized by the midwife?**

This is a similar question, again with a very practical emphasis. The key-words are 'common' and 'midwife'. The candidate who is thinking of the patient she has seen and attended is likely to give a better balanced answer than the one who is trying to visualize a page of her textbook. The second part of the question should remind the candidate that she should think primarily of potentially normal patients, for whom the midwife might reasonably be responsible.

**Q.79. Discuss the causes of delay in the second stage of labour and the recognition of these causes.**

**Q.80. What factors may affect progress in the second stage of labour?**

Questions 79 and 80 are similar, except that they are presented in general terms rather than with special reference to a particular patient.

Question 81 below is of the same type, but, again, with a slight difference of emphasis. All these questions serve to emphasize the responsibility of the midwife in the management of a hitherto normal labour.

**Q.81. What indications would lead you to send for a doctor in the second stage of labour?**

**Q.82. What is meant by the second stage of labour and how would you recognize that the patient is in this stage? Enumerate the causes of delay in this stage.** *(Scotland)*

There may, at first glance, appear to be little to write in answering this question, and certainly no adequate answer is likely to be learnt from the most diligent study of textbooks. The question is a test of clinical observation, and the student can best learn to answer it by careful, close and repeated observation of the woman in labour.

Note that, in this case the causes of delay in the second stage are only to be 'enumerated'. These, described in some detail in the answer to Question 77, have not been repeated.

**Answer.** The second stage is that period in the labour beginning at full dilatation of the cervix and ending at complete birth of the child.

The onset of the second stage of labour may be recognized as follows:

If it has not yet taken place, rupture of the membranes, occurring in a patient known to be well advanced in the first stage of labour.

A single attack of vomiting is not uncommon.

These two features are suspicious but neither universal, nor in any case diagnostic.

The next observations may be made a short time after full dilatation, when the presenting part, usually the head, has descended and now presses on the pelvic floor. This results in a change in the character of the uterine contractions, which are now described as 'expulsive'. The patient begins to 'push'. This may be recognized by the grunting noise she makes, or by the congested appearance of her face. The acute observer may well notice a slight change in the pattern of the patient's breathing, even before she is 'pushing'.

She may say she wants to 'bear down'. She may ask for a bedpan, thinking she is to have a bowel action.

A little later the anal orifice is seen to be widely dilated, with the mucosa of the anterior rectal wall visible. On palpation laterally the pressure from the presenting part is felt. (Anal dilatation alone, and without this pressure is a fallacious sign, occurring in women who attempt to hasten their labours by 'pushing' in the first stage.)

Finally the vulva gapes, and the presenting part is seen at the height of a contraction.

A patient having epidural analgesia feels neither pain nor the descending fetal head. In the absence of any urge to the patient to bear down the midwife must be, if anything, more vigilant, taking careful note of any evidence of pressure lateral to the anus.

In case of doubt, a vaginal examination may be made to ascertain that the patient is in the second stage of labour. The diagnosis is made by careful palpation, especially anterior to the presenting part as the anterior lip of the cervix is the last part to be withdrawn. If no cervix is felt the patient is in the second stage of labour, and a careful retrospective assessment may reveal the probable time of its onset.

**Q.83. How would you decide that a patient was established in the**

**second stage of labour? What are the causes of delay in this stage?**
*(Scotland)*

This question is, in many respects, similar to Question 82. Notice the minor differences in the wording.

**Q.84. Define the third stage of labour. Give the physiology and management of the normal third stage.** *(Scotland)*

If any examination question may be said to be more important, to carry more marks, to weigh more with the examiners than any other question, the distinction must go to any question about the third stage of labour. And, indeed, from a purely practical angle this is reasonable and logical. If a candidate cannot define a trisomy or locate the infundibulo-pelvic ligament or understand the mode of inheritance of spherocytosis, it is unlikely that any grave harm to mother or baby will ensue. Even if she were to misunderstand the conduct of the first or second stage of labour, the patient might well survive unscathed. But mismanagement of the third stage could all too easily lead to serious haemorrhage or even death. Here, then, are the critical questions in any midwifery examination.

Most candidates will be ready to give a good and careful answer to any question about the third stage of labour. They have been fully and repeatedly instructed in labour ward and classroom.

This question appears quite straightforward and uncomplicated: a definition, the physiology and the management in a normal case. It is probably easier to write an orderly account by describing the physiology first and then setting out the management, with references back to the physiology to demonstrate the relationship. A diagram or a series of two or three very simple diagrams will be useful.

The candidate may be anxious, knowing that there are variations in the detail of third stage management between one hospital and another; this, however, is immaterial. She should give, in full detail, the method she has been taught. Nor need she add unnecessary paragraphs about the procedures recommended by other authorities. If the candidate's account shows that she understands the method she has been taught, the examiner is prepared to accept and respect it, whether or not he agrees wholeheartedly. The basic principles are, in any case, fully agreed:

(a) to secure complete separation, descent and expulsion of the placenta and membranes, with minimum delay;

(b) to limit blood loss, both during and immediately after the third stage.

**Answer.** The third stage of labour is the stage during which the placenta and membranes separate and are expelled and haemorrhage is controlled. It lasts from the birth of the child until complete expulsion of the placenta and membranes: about 3–10 minutes.

The physiology of the third stage of labour begins during the expulsion of the fetus. Once the anterior shoulder is born a very powerful contraction with marked retraction expels the posterior shoulder, fetal trunk and legs; and the uterus is now much smaller with the fundus just below the umbilicus. This is accompanied by a marked decrease in size of the placental site which makes it impossible for the inelastic placenta to remain attached. The placenta is 'bunched' up and forced from its attachment, separation beginning as a rule in the middle.

This separation exposes some of the uterine sinuses, and a little retro-placental blood collects. This may strip off more of the placenta, thus completing its separation.

With further strong contraction and retraction the placenta is pushed downwards into the lower uterine segment or vagina, ready for expulsion; and the exposed blood-vessels of the placental site are now so firmly compressed by the 'living ligature' action of the muscle fibres surrounding them that any bleeding is effectively arrested.

Less commonly the separation begins at the edge of the placenta, no retro-placental blood collects, and the total loss is rather greater.

The third stage is terminated by expulsion of the placenta, either by the mother's own efforts, or with assistance from the midwife. The strong contraction and retraction of the empty uterus effectively controls bleeding, while more gradually, clotting occurs in the exposed blood vessels of the placental site.

*Management of the third stage.*

At the time of birth of the anterior shoulder of the fetus, the patient is given an intramuscular injection of one ampoule of Syntometrine. This contains Syntocinon 5 units and ergometrine 0·5 mg. The Syntocinon fraction will stimulate strong contraction of the uterus two and a half minutes after administration and the ergometrine will maintain continued contraction.

When the baby is born and respirations established, the cord is clamped and divided and the child warmly wrapped and put in a cot.

The mother now rests, lying on her back, with the placental end of the cord in a kidney dish at the vulva. The vulva and lower abdomen are exposed; otherwise she is warmly covered. Preferably her bladder should be almost empty. Her colour and general condition should be good: her pulse slow and of good volume.

The midwife now puts her left hand on the patient's abdomen, a sterile towel intervening. It rests on the fundus of the uterus, and must be kept absolutely still. She is ready to observe the evidence that the placenta has separated and descended to the lower segment or vagina. The uterus, already firm and hard, will shortly contract very powerfully and some or all of the following features are noted:

1. The uterus is small, round and hard, and feels somewhat like a cricket ball. This is because it is now empty and can contract very strongly.

2. The fundus is slightly higher; the uterus is now pushed up by the placenta which is now distending the lower segment and upper vagina.

3. The uterus is mobile; it is no longer anchored by the placenta.

4. The cord lengthens at the vulva; the placenta is now so much lower that more cord is visible.

A little vaginal bleeding may or may not occur. It signifies only that part, not necessarily all, of the placenta has separated.

The placenta and membranes are now withdrawn by controlled cord traction.

The midwife moves her left hand, placing it across the lower abdomen to 'hold up' the uterus and to feel its consistency (cord traction may be exerted only when the uterus is strongly contracted) while with her right hand she holds the cord firmly, close to the vulva. With her left hand holding the strongly contracted uterus, she pulls on the cord, gently but steadily, in the direction of the uterine axis; that is, towards the bed.

The placenta is felt to descend and appears at the vulva. The midwife lifts her right hand and withdraws the placenta in the direction of the vaginal axis.

She now uses her left hand to ease out the remainder of the placenta and the membranes. If the membranes are adherent they are gently eased out by twisting them into a rope. The placenta, membranes and blood, in the kidney dish, are placed on the lower shelf of the trolley for examination later.

Now, the midwife again ascertains the state of contraction of the uterus and the maternal pulse rate, noting that blood loss is minimal.

During and after the third stage a number of other features must be borne in mind:

1. A careful examination of the placenta and membranes is necessary and an attempt is made to estimate the total blood loss.

2. The patient's vulva, perineum and vaginal walls are to be inspected for lacerations. This is a convenient time for the patient to try to pass urine. Then the vulva is swabbed, a vulval pad applied, and she is made comfortable with clean linen.

3. The midwife must satisfy herself that the patient's condition is good: her colour, pulse and blood-pressure normal, her uterus well contracted and her blood loss minimal. The condition of the uterus and the blood loss should be checked at 10-minute intervals for the next hour.

4. She must satisfy herself throughout this time that the infant's colour is good, respirations are regular, and that there is no bleeding from the umbilical cord.

5. As soon as the placenta and membranes have been examined and pronounced complete, the patient may have a cup of tea. Now, too, she will be glad to see and hold her baby for a few minutes.

**Q.85. Describe the management of the third stage of labour, including a detailed account of the signs of complete placental separation.**

This question is akin to Q.84, even though the physiology, as such, is not asked. However, a 'detailed account of the signs of complete placental separation' certainly requires explanations which are related to the underlying physiology.

In her answer to Q.84, the candidate is advised to describe the particular third stage management which she has been taught. In the specimen answer (one of a number of possible answers: certainly not the only one) the signs of placental separation and descent are mentioned. This is not as contradictory as it may seem to some students. Some training schools teach one routine: others another. This, though perhaps confusing, is immaterial; the principles are common to all, namely, to shorten the third stage and to limit blood loss.

Finally, the candidate who has 'never waited for the placenta to separate' does not really lack the requisite experience. She may not have awaited these third stage changes; she has undoubtedly aided them. She has caused the cord to 'lengthen' by pulling upon it; she has made the uterus rise higher in the abdomen by pushing it upwards; and she must have noticed it becoming smaller and more mobile.

**Q.86. Describe the management of the third stage of labour.
What complications may arise?**

This question concentrates on management. The candidate may feel that, compared with the preceding ones, it is a little 'thin'. How can the answer be made more substantial?

The assumption is not really warranted. In the foregoing answers, the part dealing with management is presented fairly briefly and there is scope here for a little elaboration, particularly in respect of the observations and nursing care carried out during the hour or so after completion of the third stage.

It is worthy of note that, though, in respect of its time limits, the third stage lasts only three or four minutes, third stage management begins before the baby is completely born and does not end until about an hour after the expulsion of the placenta and membranes. The expression, 'fourth stage of labour', adopted by some authorities, has never achieved widespread popularity and it is thus all the more essential that this hour should be regarded as an extension of the third stage.

**Q.87. Describe the conduct of the third stage of labour.**
**Outline the management if excessive blood loss occurs before the delivery of the placenta.** *(Northern Ireland)*

A very similar question. Both Q.86 and Q.87 are closely related to postpartum haemorrhage questions in the next section.

# Haemorrhage

# Haemorrhage

## ANTEPARTUM HAEMORRHAGE

**Q.88. A patient, 32 weeks pregnant, is admitted to hospital with vaginal bleeding. Describe the management of this case.** *(Scotland)*

Questions on the subject of antepartum haemorrhage are asked fairly frequently in the Central Midwives Board examinations. The reason is an important practical one: that the midwife may be the first professional person to learn about this bleeding. It is no exaggeration to say that the patient's life, and that of her child, may thus depend upon the midwife's correct procedure in this emergency. It is therefore especially important that such questions should be read and interpreted correctly.

This question is simple and clear, presenting no special problems.

**Answer.** When a patient is admitted at the 32nd week of pregnancy with antepartum haemorrhage, she is kept at rest and under observation while investigations are made to determine the cause of the bleeding.

In most cases the blood loss is slight and the patient in good condition, so the investigation need not be hurried unless the bleeding becomes more severe. Meanwhile, she can be made comfortable, introduced to the other patients and she and her husband given as much reassuring information as possible.

### Investigation of vaginal bleeding

If, as is usually the case, the bleeding is slight and the patient is in reasonably good condition when first seen, she is transferred to hospital without any investigation at all.

Once the patient is in hospital the investigations would be summarized as follows:

## 1. General investigations

(a) The history is taken. If this is a booked patient the record of her pregnancy so far is noted. If she had had any previous vaginal bleeding, however slight, she would have been admitted to hospital then. She may, much earlier, have had a threatened miscarriage; in either case, this is suspicious of placenta praevia.

Antepartum haemorrhage occurs fairly often about the 32nd week; it is just possible, though rather unlikely, that the patient has had an external cephalic version performed in the last day or two. In this case there would be a possibility that the placental separation was traumatic in origin.

If the patient has essential hypertension, chronic renal disease or if she has had any indication whatever of pre-eclampsia, abruptio placentae would be suspected.

As well as the history of the pregnancy in general, that of the bleeding episode is of value. If the bleeding was entirely painless and the patient knows no cause for it, placenta praevia is suspected, though abruptio placentae with revealed haemorrhage is possible. This is likely if the onset of bleeding is related to exertion. If the patient experienced pain, there is a probability of some concealed bleeding. An attempt is made to assess the amount lost.

(b) A general examination is carried out. The patient's temperature, pulse rate and blood pressure are ascertained. A raised pulse rate would be suspicious of continuing bleeding, as would a low blood pressure. A high blood pressure is often noted in abruptio placentae and proteinuria is likely.

The haemoglobin value of the patient's blood is determined and, at the same time, two pints of blood of the correct ABO group and Rhesus type are cross-matched and set aside for use when needed.

Any evidence of labour would be noted, since the vaginal bleeding might be a heavy show at the onset of a preterm labour.

## 2. Abdominal examination

The abdomen is examined, the palpation being carried out very gently. Certain investigations yield valuable information.

(a) The state of the uterus. If it is of normal consistency and the expected size for the period of gestation and not tender, this suggests either abruptio placentae with revealed haemorrhage or placenta praevia. If it is unusually large, tense and board-like and very tender there would be some concealed haemorrhage. In this case, however, the patient would be so obviously in a state of shock that the diagnosis should be easy.

(b) The lie, the presentation and the relation of the presenting part of the pelvis. In placenta praevia of any degree, the placenta occupies space in the pelvis and, even at 32 weeks, the fetus may have an unusually high head or the presenting part may be deflected from the centre, the lie tending towards oblique.

(c) The fetal heart sounds are usually heard clearly in placenta praevia and in abruptio placentae of mild degree. In severe degrees the fetus almost always dies.

### 3. Vaginal examination

Digital examination is, for the present, to be excluded at all costs, since, if this is indeed a case of placenta praevia, the bleeding will be re-started, perhaps in more severe degree. It can then be very difficult to control.

The vulva and perineum are inspected, in order to make certain from which orifice: vagina, urethra, anus, the blood is coming. The vagina and cervix are inspected per speculum (usually after the bleeding has subsided) and any extraneous cause of vaginal bleeding is found and, if necessary, treated.

### Further investigations

It may be possible by X-ray or ultrasound scan to determine the situation of the placenta.

If placenta praevia can be excluded, either by one of these investigations, or later, by the fetal head's becoming engaged, and if bleeding has ceased, the patient may go home.

If this diagnosis is not possible, the final investigation is, if possible, delayed until the 38th week, when the fetus is sufficiently mature. This is a digital vaginal examination carried out in a theatre fully prepared for Caesarean section, the patient having a general anaesthetic, an intravenous infusion running and the cross-matched blood at hand. The obstetrician then determines if this is a case of placenta praevia and, if so, what type. If severe bleeding should occur, he carries on to an immediate Caesarean section, while a blood transfusion is given, while for Type I placenta praevia or when the placenta is not praevia, he ruptures the membranes and a Syntocinon drip infusion will probably be set up.

In severe abruptio placentae, with much concealed haemorrhage, the first essential is to replace the blood lost, and massive transfusion may be necessary. The renal function and the plasma fibrinogen must be monitored.

In rare instances when the fetal heart sounds are audible a quick Caesarean section may save the child.

More often the fetus has died. The treatment is to rupture the membranes. Usually dilatation of the cervix has already begun and labour is quickly completed.

**Q.89. Describe the management of a patient admitted at 34 weeks gestation with antepartum haemorrhage.** *(Northern Ireland)*

This question is almost precisely the same as the preceding one.

The following question, Q.90, requires that antepartum haemorrhage be defined and its causes enumerated. The emphasis here is clearly on brevity. Note also that in the second part of the question the *initial* treatment is specified. This simple word so affects the construction of an answer that the candidate is again enjoined to read and re-read the question. Some candidates find it an advantage to underline one or two words, obviously salient points, in the question. This is a good plan, provided it can be kept within reasonable limits. Over enthusiastic candidates have been known to underline every noun, verb and adjective in the question, thus reducing the all-important emphasis to nil, as W. S. Gilbert noted a hundred years ago in a well-known lyric: 'When everyone is somebodee, then no-one's anybody'.

**Q.90. Define antepartum haemorrhage and enumerate its causes.**

Describe the initial management of a patient admitted with bleeding per vaginam at the 34th week of pregnancy. *(Northern Ireland)*

**Q.91.** A multigravida has a 'show of blood' at the 38th week of pregnancy. What are the possible causes and what steps should be taken to deal with the situation?

Here is a question which has obviously been framed with great care and to help the candidate. Why (it may be asked) is 'show of blood' in quotation marks? This is to indicate that this is what the patient has described. It is perfectly possible for a multigravida who has had a blood loss of several ounces to describe it as a 'show'; just as a primigravida, more likely to become alarmed at the sight of blood, could have a 'show' of blood-stained mucus and report that she had had a haemorrhage.

## POSTPARTUM HAEMORRHAGE

Questions on the subject of postpartum haemorrhage occur fairly frequently in both the written and the oral parts of the examination. In the oral examination if the candidate's answer is not clear the examiner will obviously ask further questions. In the written part of the examination this is not possible and it is therefore all the more important that the answers shall be clearly stated.

The subject matter must be presented in good order. It is, in postpartum haemorrhage, the order of procedure which to a great extent determines its correctness; e.g. the first step is *always* to arrest the bleeding; the second to restore the patient's condition.

In this country where oxytocic drugs are given early and where midwives can give intravenous ergometrine, where the medical aid and 'flying squad' services are good, it is almost never necessary for a midwife to perform a manual removal of the placenta. The midwife may, on the other hand, practise in a primitive country where there is no doctor to help her (and incidentally no Central Midwives Board to govern and guide her). In these circumstances, if severe postpartum haemorrhage occurred and if manual removal of the placenta were really indicated she should perform this operation early, while the patient is still in reasonably good condition; not when all other measures have failed and the patient is in a state of profound shock. Too often, manual removal is considered as a last resort, and recommended (in examination papers) when all else has failed and the patient is in a state of collapse. Clearly the effect of such an operation might well be disastrous, and the examination candidate who has suggested it cannot expect to gain marks.

The answer to a question of this type must be practical. It is nearly always addressed personally to the midwife – 'what would *you* do?' 'How will *you* arrest the bleeding?' etc. – and it is up to the midwife to describe how she herself would act in this emergency.

The wording of the question should be noted with particular care. In the majority of questions it is clear whether the emergency is haemorrhage during the third stage of labour, or haemorrhage after the expulsion of the placenta.

If there is no such specification the candidate should assume that haemorrhage during the third stage is included and tackle the problem of expulsion of the placenta. Traumatic postpartum haemorrhage is a relatively unlikely contingency in a labour which is conducted by a midwife, and it need only be mentioned very briefly.

A number of questions dealing with postpartum haemorrhage are appended below. One such question is answered in full; to avoid unnecessary repetition the others are merely outlined.


**Q.92. What do you understand by postpartum haemorrhage?**
**Describe the management of a patient who has a postpartum haemorrhage immediately after the birth of her baby.**

This question is straightforward and not in any way ambiguous.

First there is a definition, and a definition should be brief, and, as the name implies definite.

The candidate who has been repeatedly enjoined to answer the question, the whole question and nothing but the question, to keep to the point and to avoid the inclusion of irrelevant material may begin to wonder if the question *is* ambiguous. Should she be defining every variety of postpartum haemorrhage? Primary? Secondary? From the placental site? From lacerations?

All these definitions would be permissible, but not essential; indeed, probably not desirable. Postpartum haemorrhage, unqualified, refers to the commonest and the most alarming variety; it calls to mind a labour ward scene: the baby just born, the mother bleeding profusely. It is used thus in conversation, in case notes, in reports and records. It means primary postpartum haemorrhage, from the placental site, immediately after the birth of the baby. All other postpartum haemorrhages are specified: secondary, traumatic, from a torn cervix, etc.

The second part of the question is entirely practical. In answering questions of this type a good and knowledgeable candidate sometimes finds herself in a quandary as, on the one hand, she aims to 'do something' for the patient, but is haunted by her responsibility to 'send for a doctor'. Which shall she put first?

No examiner enjoys reading a script wherein a patient is portrayed, bleeding profusely, while the candidate's management is set out thus: 'Send for medical aid; reassure the patient; prepare for the doctor' – and so on. The immediate reaction is – 'Why on earth doesn't she do something to stop the bleeding?' The best way out of the difficulty is probably to make a short preliminary statement, thus: 'The first essential is to stop the bleeding while at the earliest opportunity a messenger should be asked to call a doctor if there is not one present. To stop the bleeding. . . .'

**Answer.** Postpartum haemorrhage is excessive bleeding from the genital tract occurring any time after the birth of the child and up to the end of the puerperium.

By 'excessive' is meant:
(a)  an amount of more than 350 ml.
(b)  any amount (however small) which causes deterioration in the patient's condition.

The most common time for serious haemorrhage to occur is during and immediately after the third stage of labour. (Primary postpartum haemorrhage.)

The most urgent need in postpartum haemorrhage is to stop the bleeding by making the uterus contract and remain contracted. This can best be achieved by massage of the uterus – 'rubbing up a contraction' – and by giving an injection of ergometrine. If a doctor were present, he and the midwife would work together. If I were alone I should put out a call for assistance at the first opportunity, but concentrate first on controlling the haemorrhage.

Accordingly, when it became evident that the bleeding was excessive, I should immediately massage the uterus to stimulate a contraction. The patient would probably have had an intramuscular injection of Syntometrine, 1 ampoule (5 units Syntocinon and ergometrine $0 \cdot 5$ mg) at the birth of the anterior shoulder and this should stimulate good contraction of the uterus. Nevertheless, it would be wiser to repeat the oxytocic drug, so, as soon as I was able to make the uterus contract, I should administer ergometrine $0 \cdot 5$ mg intravenously. This should be done promptly, even if the child is still on the bed and the cord not divided.

When the uterus remained contracted, I should clamp and cut the cord, put the infant quickly in the cot and, returning to the mother, put my hand on the uterus to ascertain the situation of the placenta. There are two possibilities:

(a) If the uterus were high, small and mobile, and really hard, showing complete separation and descent, I should withdraw the placenta by controlled cord traction. After this I should keep my hand on the uterus, noting its consistency and massaging it if necessary, until strong contraction and retraction was sustained. Then I should note if the bladder were distended. It would be preferable not to pass a catheter, but it might be a wise precaution. If the mother were showing signs of shock with a pulse rate above 100 per minute, systolic blood pressure below 100 mm Hg, grey pallor and cold, clammy skin, I should raise the foot of the bed. The mother should be made as comfortable as circumstances permit, but with minimal disturbance. Until the placenta was examined, she should have nothing by mouth, since an anaesthetic may be needed. The state of the uterus should be kept constantly in mind and blood loss should be observed.

(b) If the uterus were broad, immobile and the fundus below the umbilicus, the placenta must still be partially attached and cannot be expelled easily. This is unimportant if the haemorrhage has been arrested, and the treatment is exactly as listed above. If, meanwhile, the placenta should separate and descend spontaneously it would be expelled as above.

Postpartum haemorrhage occurring after the completion of the third stage is easier to deal with. The management is similar to that described above, namely to 'rub up' a contraction of the uterus and to administer an oxytocic drug.

If the patient's condition had deteriorated as a result of the blood loss, urgent treatment would be necessary. The blood volume would be maintained by an intravenous dextrose infusion while blood was being cross-matched for transfusion. If the blood pressure remains low the central venous pressure and possibly the cardiac rhythm are monitored, while a massive transfusion may be necessary to reverse the shock.

On the other hand, a patient who, at the end of pregnancy, has an extra litre of circulating blood is well equipped to tolerate moderate blood loss. Not that such bleeding is desirable; but it does explain why patients remain in remarkably good condition, despite considerable blood loss. Thus, urgent treatment may not be necessary. Blood transfusion is given only in case of need. Routine haemoglobin estimation will probably reveal that the patient is anaemic and this must, of course, be corrected.

It is possible, though unlikely, that this might be a traumatic haemorrhage, and, if it were severe, it would probably arise from a deep tear of the cervix. Traumatic haemorrhage would be recognized by the fact that it continued steadily in spite of good contraction and retraction of the uterus. The treatment here would be to administer the ergometrine and expel the placenta as quickly as possible, in order to minimize bleeding from the placental site. Then, by applying fundal pressure to try to push the uterus downwards sufficiently to expose the cervix. (A speculum, if available, would facilitate this.) Direct pressure is then applied to the bleeding area, either digitally, or with sponge forceps, which could be left *in situ*.

*N.B.* If time were limited, the final paragraphs about traumatic haemorrhage could be omitted.

**Q.93. What may be the cause of excessive bleeding per vaginam immediately after the birth of the baby?**
**Describe your management of such a case.**

Here is a very similar question, having two different points: instead of a definition, the cause of this excessive bleeding is asked; and the management becomes *your* management, namely, the midwife's management. The implication here, obviously, is that the doctor is not present. It is up to the midwife to show that she will have him called without delay; but she must show, even more urgently, how she will control the haemorrhage.

**Q.94. Define primary postpartum haemorrhage and give the causes.**
**If this condition occurred, what would you do whilst awaiting the arrival of the doctor?**

This question is similar, but even more precise. Primary postpartum haemorrhage, specifically, is to be defined. The second part of the question, the emergency par excellence, is presented personally to the midwife. The doctor is on his way. Student midwives are so well prepared in this subject that they would surely acclaim the question (if not the emergency) with pleasure.

**Q.95. Describe the complications which may arise in the third stage of labour** (*Scotland*)

Since haemorrhage is the principal complication to be described, it is convenient to include this question here; but the tempo is quite different. The drama of the labour ward has given place to the drier textbook or lecture. Nevertheless, a candidate who recalls all she has seen, learned and read about postpartum collapse will be able to give the examiner some notably hair-raising reading.

**Q.96. How would you diagnose and treat haemorrhage in the third**

**stage of labour?** *(Scotland)*

This question deals only with haemorrhage occurring during the third stage. Again, the question is addressed, as it were, personally to the candidate. Whether or not it is answered in the first person is immaterial. What does matter is that the answer shall show the way in which the midwife would deal with this emergency in the absence of a doctor.

**Q.97. What natural processes prevent haemorrhage after delivery? Give the management of third stage haemorrhage.** *(Scotland)*

Here, the first part of the question deals with the very important physiology of the control of bleeding. Most candidates have learned this very thoroughly and really do understand it. The second part, unlike Question 93, asks about 'the management' – not the same in all respects as the midwife's management.

# The Puerperium

# The Puerperium

**Q.98. What are the causes of pyrexia in the lying-in period? What investigations should be undertaken?**

This is one example of a fairly common type of question dealing with the puerperium.

In order to cover the material adequately the various causes of pyrexia in the lying-in period should first be classified and then briefly described. It will be found impossible to write more than a short paragraph about each of the causes, as the answer must deal also with the investigations which are to be made and, here care is needed, as the full investigation is quite long and detailed. Order is important and the candidate should be able to recount the questions asked of the patient, the references to her previous history and the medical examination that is undertaken. For some reason the bacteriological examinations are not only clearly recalled, but all too often written first instead of last.

**Answer. The causes of pyrexia in the lying-in period.**
A. Sometimes slight pyrexia occurs where there is no infection.
1. In the so-called 'reactionary' temperature which is sometimes observed shortly after labour, and rather more especially after a labour which has been prolonged, or during which the patient has sustained trauma, the pyrexia is slight in degree and transient, the temperature settling within 24 hours of delivery.
2. Breast engorgement is sometimes associated with a slight rise of temperature to about 37·5°C. This occurs almost exclusively on the third or fourth evening after delivery.

Apart from these minor disturbances, pyrexia in the lying-in period must be considered to be due to infection of some kind.
B. Infection.
1. The commonest cause of pyrexia in the lying-in period is

urinary tract infection. It may take the form of cystitis, which is not unlikely if the patient has had urinary retention during or just after labour. Pyelonephritis is fairly common and tends to recur in patients who have had urinary tract infection during pregnancy.

2. Genital tract infection (puerperal sepsis) is a fairly common cause of pyrexia. As a rule it is a fairly mild infection, localized to the placental site and it responds quickly to the appropriate antibiotic: but sometimes it is severe, the infection spreading in the pelvis or even throughout the body, causing the patient to become seriously ill. Thrombophlebitis may occur as a complication.

3. Pyrexia during the lying-in period may be due to breast infection. This is not very common, and usually occurs during the second week after delivery. It is generally very painful, and therefore easily recognized.

4. Any pyrexial condition may arise fortuitously during the lying-in period. Examples are influenza, pneumonia or any acute specific fever. This is relatively uncommon, but should not be overlooked.

## The investigations which should be undertaken
A. History.

The patient is asked how she is feeling and is invited to report any untoward symptoms. She may feel 'off colour' or feverish; she may state specifically that she has a sore throat, severe backache, dysuria, or a pain in her leg: such symptoms require further investigation.

The patient is also asked if she is aware of having been in contact with any infection. Patients are asked to report contact with infection when they are admitted to maternity hospitals and most are careful to do so; but sometimes, in the excitement of labour, it is forgotten; and, sometimes a foreign patient has not understood clearly what she was asked. Thus, a child at home with chicken-pox may be responsible for his mother's pyrexia.

The patient's pregnancy and labour are reviewed. An attack of pyelonephritis in pregnancy may be followed by a 'flare-up' in the puerperium; a prolonged labour or a traumatic delivery can be a background to infection in the genital tract.

B. Examination of the patient.

A full medical examination may be necessary. This could include inspection of the throat, tonsils and ears and palpation of the neck glands; auscultation of the heart and lungs; examination of the breasts; palpation of the renal angles and the abdomen, including the uterus and the hypogastrium; examination of the legs; and inspection of the vulva and perineum.

C. Bacteriological Examination.

Since the two commonest causes of pyrexia in the lying-in period are urinary tract infection and genital tract infection, a high vaginal swab and a mid-stream urine specimen are always sent to the laboratory for culture and sensitivity tests. Other examinations might include a throat swab, a rectal swab, or even a blood culture.

**Q.99. What is the cause of a raised temperature in the lying-in period? What observations and investigations would help to determine the cause?**

**Q.100. Enumerate the main causes of pyrexia during the puerperium. Describe the diagnosis and treatment of one condition you mention.**

Question 99 is very similar to Question 98. Question 100, however, has a somewhat different emphasis, in which much more importance is to be attached to the latter part of the answer. Note that the diagnosis and treatment of only *one* condition is asked. It is quite easy to misread this and give a short account of *each* of the main causes of the pyrexia. This would introduce much irrelevant material, with a consequent loss of marks which is entirely unnecessary.

Which condition is to be selected? Urinary tract infection is a good choice. It is common; the candidate is probably familiar with it and can recall one or two patients so affected; and the answer is reasonably straightforward. Genital tract infection might well be chosen; but here the investigation is rather more complex and the treatment more varied. Thus, the candidate might find herself becoming side-tracked.

Breast infection is not common during the patient's stay in hospital; the numerous infections associated quite fortuitously with the early puerperium may have no obstetric relationship whatever. So these would hardly be the subjects of choice.

**Q.101. Discuss the causes of a rise of temperature in the lying-in period. What investigations are made and what are the midwife's duties?** *(Northern Ireland)*

Here is another very similar question. The causes of pyrexia can be discussed only briefly since time is needed for an account of the investigations to be undertaken.

The midwife's 'duties' are her general responsibilities as a practising midwife rather than her nursing care of the patient, and they may be conveniently summarized as Notification (inform a doctor): Isolation (of the patient herself and, possibly, of contacts) and Disinfection (depending whether or not the patient is found to have a transmissible condition).

**Q.102. A patient who had an uncomplicated labour and delivery develops a temperature of 38·6°C on the fourth day of the puerperium.**
**What are the possible causes?**
**Outline the investigations which should be made.** *(Northern Ireland)*

Here a similar problem is posed in a much more practical way. Candidates who go to the examination carrying a mental picture of a ward with its patients and their problems often prefer this phrasing. But where the question is more impersonally phrased, as are the preceding questions, candidates should appreciate that the questions are primarily practical rather than theoretical and can be put quickly into the ward rather than the textbook environment.

**Q.103. Discuss the complications which may arise during the first**

**two weeks of the puerperium.** *(Scotland)*

Question 103, on the other hand, requires a much broader review of the subject of complications of the early puerperium. It is included at this point, since infection may well constitute the commonest problem of the puerperium.

### Q.104. What difficulties may be encountered in establishing successful breast-feeding?

This is a fairly typical question about an ever-present problem. In considering an answer to this question, two main points need to be emphasized.

1. It is a 'puerperal' question, therefore the accent is to be more on the mother than on the child; though the child cannot be ignored.
2. The answer needs careful planning and, indeed, for some candidates, rigid disciplining. It is all too tempting to 'waffle' along, meandering from mother to child, from nipples to breast-milk and from pregnancy to puerperium, only to achieve an untidy, incoherent and possibly incomplete answer, which cannot be expected to give the examiner a favourable impression.

**Answer.**

A.  The breasts themselves may be, in some way, unsatisfactory.

1. The nipples may be of unsuitable shape: flat, very small, retracted or even inverted. This might have been remedied by good antenatal preparation for breast-feeding.

2. Trauma to the nipple. There may be tenderness rather than actual injury; or the nipple may be sore, oedematous, or even cracked. This is sometimes avoidable by the close supervision in the first few feeds, but it depends also on the colour and pigmentation of the nipples.

3. Excessive engorgement of the breasts. Vascular and milk engorgement will both make feeding difficult since the breast is tense and it is not easy for the child to grasp the nipple. Milk engorgement with great tension will so far disorganize the secreting function of the acini cells that lactation may fail. This can

sometimes be foreseen on the second day after delivery. Warm bathing may relieve the discomfort, but for severe engorgement the mother will need an analgesic. Most obstericians prefer not to give oestrogens.

4. Infection. Pathogenic bacteria may enter the tissues of the breast and give rise to mastitis, which in turn makes feeding difficult and painful, and, if the milk is infected, a danger to the child. Infection arising while the patient is in hospital and under constant supervision, is immediately recognized and promptly treated. Mastitis developing after her return home may continue for 24 to 36 hours before a doctor or a health visitor is consulted. It may then be too late to prevent abscess formation, with all its attendant difficulties, including the necessity to suppress lactation.

5. Insufficient secretion. This is probably the commonest single cause of failure in breast-feeding, and since it occurs most commonly when the patient is home from hospital and away from professional advice – the health visitor obviously cannot easily visit her daily – the failure may well be permanent. A vicious circle of less secretion leading to anxiety leading in turn to even less secretion will soon develop, and the anxiety is not lessened by the fretful state of the hungry child. Frequently artificial feeding is adopted.

It is difficult and, sometimes, impossible, to avoid failure of lactation. The avoidance of extreme engorgement should help. The mother should have sufficient rest and, if possible, should be freed from anxiety. Her diet should contain enough protein and she should try to drink extra milk.

B.   One of the major difficulties in establishing successful breast-feeding is inadequate sucking by the baby.

1. In the case of a preterm child who cannot attempt to feed at the breast for several weeks the mother must be very enthusiastic and energetic in her efforts to express milk regularly. All too often her milk supply is meagre and her patience insufficient.

A larger preterm child who can suck but weakly can hardly provide a good stimulus to lactation. Again, much perseverance is necessary and the mother's own natural anxiety may itself actually inhibit her lactation.

2. For some other reason, the child may not suck strongly or well: or even at all. Examples include babies with cleft palate or with a severe degree of hare lip, babies with Down's syndrome or other genetic abnormality, babies who have sustained intracranial birth trauma and babies who develop infections and become listless and anorexic.

3. Sometimes a perfectly normal baby, strong and healthy, will refuse to suck at the breast, but will take hungrily a feed given by spoon or bottle.

C.   The difficulty may lie in the attitude of the mother, or even of the father.

The mother can, though starting with the best intentions, become discouraged if her baby is not enthusiastic about the first few feeds. In a hospital where the staff are able to give her much help and encouragement during this time, the problem may be overcome. The other patients may help, an experienced multigravid neighbour often supplying the necessary continued reassurance. Conversely, a discouraged young woman who sees a neighbouring patient bottle-feeding with apparent ease and success, may well be persuaded to abandon her efforts and follow this example.

Finally, there are husbands and wives who hold diametrically opposed views about breast-feeding and who do not come to terms with the problem before the child is born. The woman who wishes to breast-feed is not at all likely to make progress if she knows her husband is opposed to the idea. Nor, if she herself does not wish to breast-feed, is she likely to succeed if she is merely reluctantly falling in with her husband's wishes.

Thus, the difficulties that may be encountered in the establishment of breast-feeding include those related to the breast and its secretion, the failure of the child to suck adequately, and the problems experienced by the mother in relation to her hospital environment, her family or herself.

**Q.105. Describe the changes which take place in the breast during pregnancy. What anatomical abnormalities of the breast make breast-feeding difficult? How can you deal with these?**

In this question, after an account of physiological changes in the breast, the candidate needs to select the anatomical abnormalities which can present difficulties.

**Q.106. Discuss the measures that can be taken during pregnancy and the puerperium to promote successful breast-feeding.**

**Q.107. What can be done during pregnancy and after delivery to help the establishment of breast-feeding.**

Questions 106 and 107 are straightforward. No complicated preparation is required, but the candidate should prepare an orderly plan and stick to it. The same applies to Question 108, below.

**Q.108. Describe the anatomy of the female breast. Discuss the management of excessive fullness of the breasts in the early days of lactation.**

**Q.109. How would you recognize retention of urine during the first week of the puerperium?**
**State briefly what may be the causes.**

The answer to this very practical question may be learned from observation of patients in the lying-in period rather than from textbooks. Retention of urine is by no means uncommon during this period, and the responsibility for detecting it rests almost entirely upon the midwife. Questions of this type offer considerable scope to the student midwife who finds theoretical work difficult, but who learns readily from practical experience.

**Answer.** Any or all of the following observations would lead me to think that a woman was not completely emptying her bladder:
1. The amount of urine passed. (It is a wise precaution routinely to measure, or to ask the patient to measure, the amount of urine

passed in the first 48 hours after delivery.) There is a marked diuresis in the early lying-in period, and the daily excretion commonly amounts to 2·5 litres. The passage of this quantity would not, of course, be any guarantee that the patient's bladder was empty, but the converse – a total output of appreciably less – would raise my suspicions. Similarly, failure to pass urine within six hours of delivery, irrespective of the amount of fluid drunk, would be suspicious.

2. Displacement of the fundus uteri. If at any time the fundus appeared higher than would be expected; or, even more typically, if it were displaced upwards and to the right side, the probable cause would be a full bladder.

3. Palpation of the bladder. The most valuable evidence that the bladder is not empty is to palpate it directly. During the first few days after delivery the lower abdomen should always be palpated as soon as possible after the patient has passed urine. If the bladder can be felt as a soft fluctuant swelling then it most certainly is not empty.

Symptoms are not reliable in the lying-in period.

The patient may or may not report that she has failed to pass urine. She may have passed some urine but retained a good deal more, and be unaware of this; and, typically, she will not complain of pain or discomfort from an over-distended bladder. The abdominal wall is so lax that often discomfort is not experienced.

Retention of urine can thus be overlooked, and as it continues the patient might now complain of increased frequency, and the passage of small quantities of urine. This is an indication that the bladder is greatly distended with a small overflow at intervals. It can be avoided by careful observation and earlier recognition and treatment of the retention.

Pain would be a late symptom, due, not only to the retention of urine, but to an infection of the urinary tract which had now developed.

The causes of retention of urine in the early postnatal period are numerous. The retention may be absolute, it may be the retention of some residual urine in the bladder, or, if this is overlooked, it may progress to retention with overflow.

The first and simplest cause may be the strangeness of the whole procedure when first experienced by a hospital patient. For a patient who must stay in bed and use a bedpan, the bedpan itself, the unaccustomed posture and the lack of privacy in a hospital ward all contribute to difficulty. Retention of urine is uncommon in most patients who get up and go to the lavatory.

The patient may be inhibited further by fear: fear of dysuria, fear of 'straining' lest she break the sutures in her perineum. The pain itself may be very real, especially after a traumatic delivery, while sometimes the necessity for catheterization during labour seems to aggravate a tendency to retention.

Finally, as mentioned above, the patient may not realize that her bladder is distended, since the laxity of her abdominal muscles means that she experiences no discomfort.

**Q.110. What disorders of micturition may occur in the puerperium? Describe the management of each.**

**Q.111. What disturbances of micturition may occur in the lying-in period. Give the management of one of these.**

Questions 110 and 111 are similar, both rather different from Question 109 in that they deal with disturbances of micturition other than retention of urine. In question 110 the management of all these conditions is to be described, albeit briefly; but in Question 111, only *one* is to have its management described. The obvious choice would be retention of urine.

**Q.112. What are the causes of retention of urine in the puerperium?**
**How is this condition diagnosed and how can it be treated?**
*(Northern Ireland)*

A very similar question. The order is changed and a little more material is required. The time limit being the same, the inference is that rather less detail is needed.

**Q.113. What urinary tract complications may occur in the puerperium? Indicate briefly how these may be avoided and treated.**

Question 113 covers much more material. The candidate is advised to notice carefully the difference between disturbance or disorder of *micturition* and complications involving the *urinary tract*. Questions 110 and 111 would not include pyelonephritis. Question 113 certainly would.

# The New-born Child

# The New-born Child

In both the written and the oral part of the examination, questions about low birth-weight babies occur quite frequently. This is hardly surprising; preterm and other small babies present one of our greatest problems; and their survival is closely enough related to the quality of the nursing care they receive.

Here is a typical and recurrent question.

**Q.114. Describe the care of a preterm baby.**

**Answer.** There are four principal objectives in the care of a preterm baby.
1. The establishment and maintenance of respiration.
2. The prevention of infection.
3. The provision of the best environment, chiefly to maintain body temperature.
4. The provision of a suitable diet.

1. The baby may have lungs which are fairly well developed, but the respiratory centre is immature and the respiratory muscles weak. After initial gentle resuscitation, a baby weighing about 1500 g should be put in an incubator, the temperature being 32°–34°C and the relative humidity 75 per cent. If the child is at all cyanotic, extra oxygen should be given without hesitation, since it is clearly needed; if his colour is already good, extra oxygen is not only unnecessary, but dangerous, so it is avoided. In case the air passages become blocked, a suction apparatus should be at hand. The child needs to be watched closely.
2. Preterm babies are exceptionally vulnerable to infection, and should be nursed in a special care baby unit isolated from almost everyone except their own attendants. Visiting of any preterm

infant should be restricted to the parents, who should be gowned and masked in the same way as the attendants and who, like the attendants, should be free from infection of any kind.

Linen and equipment brought into contact with the child should, if possible, be autoclaved, attendants need to pay very strict attention to hand-washing and domestic staff must be fully instructed about the cleaning and disinfecting of the room.

Many authorities recommend the administration of a prophylactic antibiotic where there is an increased risk of respiratory tract infection. This would apply particularly to babies with respiratory distress syndrome.

3. A baby who cannot maintain a normal body temperature should be nursed in an incubator having, as described above, a temperature of 32°–34°C. Even so, the rectal temperature which is taken twice daily, is often subnormal, possibly only 34°–35°C at first. When, after a week, or two, the heat-regulating centre begins to function, the child's temperature will gradually rise to 36° or 36·5°C and now, other factors being satisfactory, the infant may be moved from the incubator to a warm cot in a well-heated room, its temperature 21°–24°C.

At first, the atmosphere should be kept at a high relative humidity, since this may aid respiration, while it conserves body heat by lessening fluid loss via the skin. It is an advantage, too, that fluid loss is avoided.

The baby should be disturbed as little as possible, so that washing and cleaning is cut down to the barest minimum, the genitalia being cleaned when necessary with sterile liquid paraffin. While it is true that as little handling as possible is desirable, it must be borne in mind at the same time that rigid exclusion from all human contact may, in fact, do psychological harm and the baby who is taken out of his incubator for some feeds and cuddling will derive a feeling of security from this contact with the nurse and as soon as possible his mother.

4. Feeding is a particular problem, since, though the child is growing and developing fast and needs, in relation to his weight, more food than a term infant, his ability to take food, to suck, swallow and digest, is extremely limited. Accordingly, small frequent feeds are introduced soon after birth and increased gradually as the child seems able to take more, though it may be two or

three weeks before the full caloric requirement is reached.

If possible, expressed breast milk, either the mother's or from a bank, is given. The daily intake should increase from approximately 60 ml per kg on the first day to 200 ml per kg by the end of a fortnight. For very small babies, who cannot suck or swallow, tube feeds are necessary. Once the infant begins to suck and swallow, bottle feeding can be introduced gradually. Eventually, the baby can take all his feeds by bottle, or even, if the mother has maintained her milk supply, from the breast.

**Q.115. Describe the management of a preterm infant.** *(Scotland)*

This is almost identical with Q.114.

**Q.116. Describe the care of a baby delivered at 36 weeks where the mother is suffering from diabetes.** *(Scotland)*

In Question 116, the preterm baby of a diabetic mother presents a number of special problems, though in fact simple care of the preterm baby constitutes an important part of the answer.

**Q.117. What are the differences between a preterm and a small-for-dates baby? Give the basic principles in the management of each.** *(Scotland)*

A straightforward question, the first part of which requires that a number of features be compared and contrasted. If three or four characteristics are to be compared, a series of paragraphs is sufficient, thus:

A preterm baby is one who is born before the 37th week of pregnancy, whereas a small-for-dates baby is one whose birth weight falls below the 10th centile for gestational age.

The preterm baby has a reddish skin, whereas . . . . . , continuing for the necessary number of paragraphs.

Even so, it has already become a time-wasting and repetitive exercise. To continue thus, contrasting a dozen different features would be merely absurd, creating in the candidate a situation of wrist-aching exhaustion and in the examiner one of crashing boredom.

It is very much quicker and simpler to set out a table on the lines of that on p. 145. Moreover, if, during her earlier studies, the candidate has noted that there are twelve comparable characteristics she will not so easily forget any essentials when she comes to recall her table. As in Q.30, it is recommended that the table should be spread right across a double page of the script.

Should the second part of the answer (it might be asked) be set out similarly? This would certainly be possible; but it might become a little too ponderous and an alternative arrangement is suggested.

*Management.* There are four basic principles in the management of preterm babies.

1. To establish and maintain respiration. With very small babies, in whom respiratory distress syndrome is a particular hazard, many difficulties may be encountered.

2. To develop a satisfactory feeding régime. The first need is to start with human milk, which is life-saving; the second, to give small, frequent, gradually increasing feeds, probably by naso-oesphageal tube.

3. To provide an appropriate environment. This includes warmth, high humidity, oxygen when necessary; also gentle handling, skill and dexterity in all observation checks and nursing procedures; and the watchfulness and sixth sense of the specialist.

4. To protect the infant from infection. This, too, is a matter of round-the-clock vigilance, together with a rigid aseptic and antiseptic discipline on the part of everyone entering the special care unit.

In the management of the small-for-dates baby, these same principles may be applied, but here with a difference of emphasis.

1. It may not be easy to initiate a satisfactory respiratory pattern, but once this is achieved, there is no problem.

2. The need here is early feeding, extra dextrose to prevent hypoglycaemia, and generous amounts of food. Human milk is desirable, but not usually essential. The child will probably be hungry and suck avidly.

3. This principle applies with equal force. The small-for-dates

| Classification | Preterm Baby | Small-for-Dates Baby |
|---|---|---|
| | Born before 37th week | Weight below 10th centile for gestational age |
| Skin | Reddish pink, lanugo + | Dry, wrinkled, scaly |
| Vernix | Present, often abundant | Usually absent or scanty |
| Cranial bones | Soft, mobile, wide sutures | Hard, well ossified |
| Subcutaneous fat | Scanty | Scanty |
| Abdomen | Protuberant | Scaphoid |
| Umbilical cord | Firm, fairly thick | Thin, yellowish, flaccid |
| Activity | Minimal, lies in 'frog' attitude | Usually active, flexed attitude |
| Reflexes | Sucking and swallowing poor | Sucking and swallowing good |
| Muscle tone | Poor to fair | Fair to good |
| Cry | Weak, whining | Usually mature, vigorous |
| Special problems | Respiratory distress syndrome Hypothermia Intraventricular haemorrhage | Hypoglycaemia Hypocalcaemia Hypothermia |

This table sets out a number of well-defined contrasting features; but, often the distinction is much less clear-cut, since preterm babies are not infrequently small-for-dates in addition. This is not usually of practical importance, however, as there are so many similarities in the management in both groups.

baby is ready to be transferred to a cot earlier than his preterm counterpart.

4. This ruling applies without exception, to all special care babies, of whatever size or maturity.


**Q.118. What is: (a) a prematurely born (preterm) baby? (b) a light-for-dates baby?**
   **Describe the complications which may occur in each.** *(Scotland)*

Though this answer is based on practically the same material as Q.117, the approach is entirely different. These two types of low birth-weight baby are to be clearly defined and the major part of the answer is to be an account of the complications to which they are prone.

The next two questions, both concentrating on small-for-dates babies, ask about complications.


**Q.119. What factors are associated with a small-for-dates fetus during pregnancy? How would you recognize a dysmature baby at birth? What complications may occur? Describe their treatment.**


**Q.120. Describe the care of a baby delivered at 39 weeks gestation, weighing 1800 grams. What are the main complications that may occur?**

The candidate will have noticed the various terms in current use to describe a baby that is below the expected gestational size. The whole concept is a relatively recent one; no standard nomenclature has yet been adopted. It is true that the term 'dysmature' is used rather less now than in 1972, when Q.119 was set. Small for dates, with or without hyphens, has the advantage that it can be used to describe the fetus as well as the neonate. Light for dates is more precise. Whatever the designation, the candidate will be familiar with the appearance and behaviour of these babies and it is principally this clinical experience which provides the material for her answer.


**Q.121. Describe the management of a baby with an Apgar score of 4 at one minute after delivery.** *(Scotland)*

Questions on the subject of low Apgar score, asphyxia and resuscitation at birth are commonly asked in the course of the examinations. This is understandable since this is one of the emergencies with which the midwife may have to deal. While it is true that medical assistance is, as a rule, readily available, the fact remains that, in this country, in three-quarters of all deliveries the midwife is the most senior person present. Her responsibilities are considerable and it is reasonable that the examination should take account of this.

In answering questions about this emergency many marks are lost quite unnecessarily, not through inadequate knowledge, but as a result of lack of thought and attention to elementary principles. These principles (which may equally well be applied in any circumstances of asphyxia such as recovery from anaesthesia, eclamptic fits, or even drowning) are simple.

Firstly, it is necessary to secure and maintain a clear airway.

Secondly, and in this order, oxygen must be provided.

Thirdly, and throughout the case, quiet and warmth are essential.

**Answer.** The first aim is to clear the air passages of liquor amnii, mucus, blood, meconium, or any other foreign material.

It is reasonable to assume that up to one minute after birth routine care has been given, namely, that when the child's head was born mucus was wiped from the nose and mouth; and that immediately after birth a mucus extractor was used to clear the mouth, pharynx and nostrils of mucus and any other material which might block the airway.

With an Apgar score of only 4 one minute after birth, the attendant will quickly complete the clamping and dividing of the cord, so that the infant can be rapidly placed on a warmed resuscitation table, lying flat, and with the head to one side. It may be necessary to continue the attempts to clear the pharynx of mucus.

Secondly, oxygen should be given as quickly as possible.

If the child gasps occasionally, oxygen may be given through a soft plastic funnel over the nose and mouth. For this purpose the oxygen may be given at 1 to 2 litres per minute, and even with the faintest respiratory gasps some oxygen will be absorbed.

If the child makes no attempt to breathe it is necessary to try to introduce oxygen by some means.

(a) The doctor, or the midwife, if she is instructed could pass a small laryngoscope and introduce an endotracheal tube past the vocal cords. Then, by suction, he could extract mucus which might be blocking the trachea. After this, he would give oxygen intermittently at a positive pressure of 30 cm water. This intermittent positive pressure respiration, because it actually introduces oxygen into the lungs, is the most satisfactory way to deal with a severely asphyxiated baby, whose primary need is to have oxygen circulating in the blood and reaching the respiratory centre.

Whichever way the oxygen is given, some will circulate in the blood and reach the vital centres in the medulla oblongata, and gradually restore their failing function.

The more quickly the cardiac and vasomotor centres recover, the more quickly will the child's circulation and condition improve. At the same time the respiratory centre will recover and regular respirations will be established.

(b) In emergency, and in the absence of better facilities either doctor or midwife could administer mouth to mouth respiration (the 'kiss of life'). With the attendant's mouth over the baby's mouth, air is blown in, in short intermittent puffs. Some should enter the upper respiratory tract and could reach the lungs. If oxygen were available the midwife could put the oxygen tube in her mouth and thus puff the released oxygen into the baby's mouth.

The other essentials are warmth, rest, and gentle handling during the whole of this time, and close observation for at least 48 hours afterwards. Warmth, because all newly-born babies, emerging from the intra-uterine warmth to a much lower temperature, become very readily cold. This is particularly the case in an infant whose circulation is poor. Rest is essential because in severe asphyxia the child is in a condition of circulatory failure comparable to shock, which is worsened by unnecessary disturbance. The handling of the child is to be as little and as gentle as possible, again, not to worsen the shock; and also because in severe asphyxia there is always a possibility that the child has sustained some intracranial trauma and needs to be kept very quiet. It is for this reason, too, that, as soon as the air passages are clear, the child should be laid flat rather than kept with the head lowered.

When breathing appears to be established the baby can be put into an incubator and transferred to the special care baby unit. If the respiratory rate becomes regular and the child's condition improves, the oxygen can be discontinued but he should remain under close observation for 48 hours.

If respirations continue irregular and shallow, it will be necessary to monitor the blood gases ($pO_2$ and $pCO_2$) in order to discover the degree of metabolic acidosis. To correct this an infusion of dextrose 10 per cent with sodium bicarbonate $8\cdot4$ per cent can be given via the umbilical vein.

It is possible that the child's failure to breathe is related to the recent administration of pethidine to the mother. If this is clearly the case, but not in any other circumstances, it might be considered advisable to administer Neonatal Lethidrone (nalorphine) $0\cdot25$ mg intramuscularly or into the umbilical vein. This drug quickly reverses the respiratory depressant effect of pethidine, which can be transmitted from the mother, via the placenta, to the fetus. However it is not easy to be certain that the respiratory depression is definitely related to the mother's pethidine.

**Q.122. Describe the management of a baby who fails to breathe at birth.** *(Northern Ireland)*

This question, though differently phrased, is so similar that the same answer would suffice.

**Q.123. An infant 3 minutes after birth is pale, limp, has not yet made any inspiratory effort and has a heart rate of 80 beats per minute.**
   **What are the likely causes of such a condition?**
   **What action should the midwife take?**

Here the candidate is invited to translate the clinical picture into an Apgar score of 2 or 3. This, 3 minutes after birth, is rather gloomier than in the preceding question, but the pattern is the same; the resuscitation of a baby born in poor condition.

There is, however, a slight shift of emphasis: the likely causes are to be reviewed, while the management is restricted to the midwife's action.

**Q.124. What are the causes of intra-uterine hypoxia?**
**Describe the principles underlying the management of severe asphyxia in the newborn.** *(Scotland)*

The resemblance to the two preceding questions is inescapable; but here, since the candidate is asked to describe principles rather than details of management, it may be inferred that the second part of the answer will be quite brief; and, as a corollary, that the background to intra-uterine hypoxia should be considered more fully.

**Q.125. How can fetal hypoxia be diagnosed during labour? Write an account of the resuscitation of an asphyxiated baby.** *(Northern Ireland)*

Here, however, the emphasis is on the recognition of fetal hypoxia. This excellent question helps the candidate to appreciate the close relationship between the fetal and neonatal condition.

**Q.126. A newborn infant fails to breathe. What may cause this, and what would you do?** *(Northern Ireland)*

This question is very similar to Q.124, though rather less precise. As the possible cause of the child's failure to breathe has to be considered, the management (by the midwife: 'what would *you* do?') would necessarily be rather less detailed.

**Q.127. What examination would you make of a newly born baby?
Give your reasons.**

Here is a personal question, directed immediately to the candidate and emphasizing the midwife's responsibility, both to her
medical colleagues and to the baby's mother and father.

As always, the phrasing of the question should be noted. At first
glance, it is uncomplicated enough: an account of the actual
procedures; then an explanation of the purpose.

This kind of question has, over the years, been set often enough
for experienced examiners to make some assessment of candidates' thinking, as they planned their answers.

Over-cautious candidates have sometimes seen two questions:
first the examination; then the reasons. With the best possible
intentions, they have written long and repetitious answers, wasting their own and their examiners' time and gaining no extra
credit; indeed perhaps losing marks, in that the remainder of the
paper would necessarily be more hurried and perhaps less accurate. No; each particular investigation, described and explained,
makes for a much simpler and clearer answer.

Secondly, the candidate is urged to be practical and to think of
the labour ward scene in planning her answer. If the child has a
complete hare lip or a large meningocele, this is only too obvious
at the moment of birth; the shocked silence and the mother's
awareness of the atmosphere are all too eloquent. Less obvious
defects are thought of as the child comes under constant observation, during the next half hour. 'Does that baby look mongoloid or
is it my imagination?' one hears a doctor or midwife ask a colleague: a doubt that is to be confirmed or refuted later. Yet
candidates have been noted to conjure up a picture of carefully
studying the appearance of the child in the cot and thoughtfully
making a diagnosis of anencephaly.

**Answer.** The first examination of a newly-born baby is carried out
as soon after birth as is reasonably possible, often in the delivery
room.

The sooner an apparently healthy baby can be examined in
detail, the sooner can this probable healthy state be confirmed.
On the other hand, if there should be an unsuspected defect, the

earlier this is brought to light the better. Treatment can be started earlier – a life-saving measure in such conditions as oesophageal atresia; and no false hopes are raised in the mother's mind, thence to be broadcast to her husband and relatives.

The general appearance of the child, with a good pink colour and regular respirations, is being noted frequently. The Apgar score is probably 8 or more.

A systematic head to foot examination has advantages. It ensures that no visible defect shall be overlooked and it avoids undue exposure of the child to chilling.

The head is examined first. The shape is noted, slight moulding and a small caput being normal. Familiarity with the normal size of the head in relation to the trunk means that microcephaly or a mild degree of hydrocephalus would be suspected, while prominent scalp veins tend to support the latter feature. When the face is looked at, deviations from normal, such as mongoloid features, micrognathia and the lopsided appearance in facial palsy, will be seen.

It is better to inspect the baby's eyes whenever he opens them than to try to force the lids apart, a deviation from routine that is well worth while. Only rarely is microphthalmia found; nystagmus is common and, in an otherwise normal baby, probably of no import. Small sub-conjunctival haemorrhages are also common, disperse quickly and cause no anxiety in the attendants; the mother may be worried at the sight of blood and need reassurance. Small red patches over the eyelids and on the back of the neck ('stork bites'), similarly disappear quickly. The ears are usually normal, but small skin tags, anterior to the ear, are sometimes seen and may be associated with abnormal development of the mandible. Low set ears should be noted on account of their association with renal and other abnormalities.

The mouth is inspected in a good light, conveniently when the baby cries. A hare lip is hardly to be overlooked, but the hard and soft palates and uvula must be seen to be normal. Occasionally a lower incisor tooth has erupted; this is unimportant. Undue drainage of mucus is suspicious of oesophageal atresia.

Only now is the baby unwrapped.

The neck is inspected. A sternomastoid haematoma is rarely seen so early. Very rarely are the short neck found in the

Klippel-Feil syndrome and the loose skin folds in Turner's syndrome seen.

The respiratory movements are noted. Sternal recession is unlikely in a healthy mature baby.

When the abdomen is inspected, undue distension, possibly due to some type of intestinal obstruction, might be seen. Umbilical hernia is not common though a protruding umbilicus is seen often enough, especially in babies of the West African and Caribbean ethnic group. The cord vessels are counted; three is normal. If only two are present the child may have a renal defect.

The genitalia usually reveal the sex clearly enough. Sometimes, however, a large clitoris may be difficult to distinguish from a penis, or a bifid scrotum from labia majora. In these cases of intersex, early investigation is important.

In baby boys, the scrotum is examined to determine if the testes have descended, and the exact location of the urinary meatus is noted. Hypospadias is uncommon and epispadias relatively rare, but they should not be overlooked. It is unnecessary at this juncture to try to retract the foreskin.

The legs are examined next, the checks being for free movement and a standard test to exclude congenital dislocation of the hip. The ankles are carefully examined. Mild positional talipes is common and easily corrected by prompt treatment. Severe degrees are easily seen. The feet are examined, the toes being counted and any webbing noted. The plantar creases, an index to maturity and normality, are also observed.

The baby is now turned over and lies prone, head to one side, while his back is examined. A finger, run down the spine, can detect any irregularity in the spinous processes of the vertebrae. A growth of hair over the sacral area is suspicious of spina bifida occulta, while a dimple, low down in this area suggests a pilonidal sinus. Usually the patency of the anus is checked by gently passing an oiled catheter. Some authorities omit this examination if the child has passed meconium.

If, as is usual, no abnormality is found, the mother is informed promptly. If, on the other hand, any suspicious feature comes to light the baby is seen by a paediatrician.

Weighing, measuring and the initial cleaning and dressing of the baby may well be deferred for an hour or two.

**Q.128. Give a detailed description of the routine examination of a newborn baby.** *(Scotland)*

**Q.129. Describe the routine examination of a newborn infant to detect congenital abnormalities.** *(Northern Ireland)*

Although the material in these two questions is similar to that in the foregoing one, the phrasing is somewhat different and one has to wonder whether the appropriate answer, too, would differ greatly.

A careful analysis of possible answers shows that this is not so. True, there is a shift of emphasis; but giving reasons for the procedure is merely explaining its purpose. Describing an examination in greater detail does much, in fact, to explain its purpose.

The foregoing answer, whether slightly modified or not, is one possible way of dealing with both questions.

**Q.130. What factors predispose to intracranial injury of the newborn? Describe the management of a baby with this condition.** *(Scotland)*

A little thought is needed in order to make as clear a distinction as possible between predisposing factors and causes. A predisposing factor makes an event more likely to occur; a cause actually initiates the event. Thus high parity is a factor which predisposes to postpartum haemorrhage. Many women having a fifth or sixth or even a tenth child do not have a postpartum haemorrhage; but they are all at more than average risk. One of them, *or* a primigravida *does* have a postpartum haemorrhage; the cause (whatever the parity) is failure of the uterus to contract strongly enough.

**Answer.** One of the most important factors predisposing to intracranial injury of the newborn is hypoxia: both the fetal and neonatal types. The low pH value of the blood is associated with marked venous congestion and haemorrhages readily occur.

The preterm baby is similarly at risk by virtue of the soft, mobile, easily squeezed cranial bones and the fragility and consequent vulnerability of the soft tissues. Less commonly the abnormal types of moulding associated with cephalopelvic disproportion, persistent occipitoposterior and breech delivery contribute to this trauma.

*Management.* At birth, neonatal hypoxia is to be reversed as quickly as possible. Intravenous sodium bicarbonate raises the blood pH and some authorities recommend the administration of Konakion (Vitamin $K_1$) 1 mg, which could help to reduce haemorrhage.

After resuscitation, the baby is transferred to an intensive care baby unit. Here respirations and, if necessary, temperature, pulse and blood pressure can be continuously monitored.

Meanwhile, the most essential feature of the care of this baby is absolute quiet. Handling is reduced to a minimum, weighing, measuring and cleaning being deferred. Feeding is by indwelling oesophageal tube, small frequent feeds of expressed breast milk being given up to a total amount calculated on the child's apparent weight and maturity.

Some of these babies remain inert and limp; others manifest marked irritability, sometimes with convulsions. For the latter, such drugs as diazepam $0 \cdot 1$ mg/kg b.d. or t.d.s. may be prescribed: occasionally, phenobarbitone or even chloral hydrate are used. Oxygen is given as needed.

Many apparently well babies come into a 'suspect' class by reason of slightly suspicious behaviour. This may include refusal or inability to suck, crying or screaming when feeding is attempted, unexplained vomiting, fretfulness and wakefulness. Such babies should be watched very closely and treated as cases of intracranial trauma until there is no longer any evidence that this is the case.

All affected babies should be brought to a specialist follow-up clinic for two years.

**Q.131. What are the signs of intracranial trauma in a newborn infant? Describe the management.** *(Scotland)*

This question approaches the same subject in a somewhat more practical way. The candidate may well spend time giving as full an account as she can of the clinical picture. A clear and orderly description from which the examiners can readily visualize the baby will gain marks. The second part is the same as in Q.130, with one reservation: if the clinical picture is not asked, it may still be necessary to refer to it obliquely in connection with treatment. Thus in Q.131 it might be necessary to steer away from obvious repetition.

### Q.132. What are the causes of intracranial birth injury? What is the clinical picture and how is the baby nursed?

Here is the third approach. The causes will need to be covered quite briefly, again leaving time for the presenting of an adequate clinical picture. Finally, the candidate must ask herself how nursing differs from management. While it may be necessary to refer to the medical care, this should be rather outlined than given in full.

# Community Health

# Community Health

Candidates looking through old examination papers will notice, perhaps with surprise, that the same question may be asked in the First Examination (now discontinued) and the Integrated Examination. 'Describe the anatomy of the pregnant uterus at term', 'Discuss current methods of relief of pain in labour', 'Discuss the management of pre-eclampsia in a primigravida 32 weeks pregnant'. Further investigation discloses this same question appearing in Midwife Teachers Diploma examination papers.

It is not, of course, the question so much as the answer that matters. A candidate who has completed twelve months' training is expected to give a broader and more knowledgeable answer than one who has had only six months' training. The experienced midwife's answer is altogether more informed and mature.

The Integrated Examination paper, however, has one kind of question that would never have been set in a First Examination, namely, a question needing an answer which draws upon community experience. A few such questions are considered below, some from midwifery and some from Community Health papers.

## Q.133. Discuss the advantages and disadvantages of home confinement.

Though for many years there has been a steady increase in the numbers of women both seeking and being advised hospital confinement, the issue remains controversial; and, in this question, the word 'discuss' invites argument pro and con.

It is almost impossible to answer such a question other than in essay form. Many candidates dislike these essay-type questions and often they are answered in a series of statements. This is usually sufficient to show the examiner that the candidate has acquired a grasp of the subject; but it does deviate somewhat from what is asked. With a little practice most candidates should be able to achieve an essay which is adequate. Outstanding literary merit is neither asked nor expected.

To a candidate writing in a foreign language the difficulty is even greater; and indeed, most English candidates would blench at the idea of writing an essay in Urdu or Mandarin. However, examiners are sympathetic people; and good foreign candidates get their material 'across' successfully.

One final point: many of these essay-type questions occur in Part 1 of the Community Health paper, in which two questions out of the three set are to be answered. It is often possible to avoid the detested discussion.

**Answer.** Although nowadays few women choose to have a home confinement, it does offer certain advantages over a confinement in hospital. It is true that most of these advantages are of a domestic or social nature and relatively few concerned with the health and safety of mother and baby. Nevertheless, social and domestic factors weigh heavily with some women and, within limits of safety, these views are to be respected.

One major advantage is that the mother, though hardly able personally to run the house for a week or two, keeps her place as conductor of the family orchestra. The disruption of a united family by the mother's admission to hospital can be extremely disturbing and many mothers wish ardently to avoid it. Even though she ceases cleaning and cooking for a few days, she is there, for the most part accessible to husband and children, advising the home help and generally controlling the household. Young children can stay at home rather than be sent to relatives and schoolchildren are seen off and greeted on their return. Whether a home help from the Social Services Department is employed, a relative comes to stay, or the husband takes time off from work to act as home help, the important fact is that a break-up, however temporary, in the family unit is avoided. Moreover, the baby is accepted by all from the time of birth. The mother cannot easily become obsessed with the care of this new baby, to the chagrin and distress of the other children. Particularly is a young 'ex-baby' happier and less likely to develop a pattern of jealousy.

The mother receives good continuity of care. Together with the general practitioner obstetrician, one midwife will be in attendance, with a second – possibly a third, paying occasional visits. She has probably met them all in the antenatal period and knows them well. The same applies to the health visitor who 'takes over' from doctor and midwife.

Home confinement probably permits easier sleep, rest and relaxation. Hospital patients, even those in single rooms, often find their rest disturbed by other mothers' babies; a hospital mother whose baby is fretful is herself fearful that he will disturb other patients. The hospital day has become much more relaxed and informal in recent years; but, of necessity, the day starts early and continues busy. A mother at home can give her baby an early feed and settle down to sleep again. Finally, hospital catering comes in for a good deal of adverse criticism, some of it certainly justifiable. It is not surprising that many women prefer the meals they have at home.

These simple domestic details may, in themselves, seem trivial; but their psychological value is considerable and, in an extreme case, loss of this security could well be a contributory factor to puerperal psychosis.

The baby, too, may well partake in this security. It does appear that breast feeding is established more easily and with a greater measure of success, a fact we are coming to appreciate more and more.

In considering the disadvantages of home confinement, the outstanding factor is the loss in physical safety. Though home delivery has the psychological advantage, the statistically established risks preclude it for all but a chosen few.

The list of contra-indications is almost endless: all primigravidae; an obstetric history ranging from pre-eclampsia to postpartum haemorrhage, from hydramnios to forceps delivery, from stillbirth to preterm labour. It is easier to be positive. Women suitable for home confinement are under 35, healthy, and have had one or two completely normal confinements; and their current pregnancies continue uncomplicated. The home should be suitable and the patient should wish to be confined there.

All this applies to a fairly small number of women. Numbers diminish when some of them are found to have or to develop a complication decreeing that the place of confinement shall be reconsidered. Obvious examples are twin pregnancy, pre-eclampsia and antepartum haemorrhage.

More unfortunately, after a normal pregnancy, a complication of labour may necessitate transfer to hospital. This is disturbing enough in the first stage; in the second stage it must be very traumatic to all concerned; and perhaps all for a simple 'lift-out' which, for the hospital patient, creates only minimal disturbance.

The worst hazard in a home confinement is probably postpartum haemorrhage, with or without a retained placenta. High risk patients are diverted to hospital; but there are no 'no risk' patients. Any labour may be complicated by postpartum haemorrhage. It is for this emergency above all others that the 'Flying Squads' exist. It is with postpartum haemorrhage in mind that many authorities advocate 100 per cent hospital delivery.

Though the community midwife stays with the patient throughout labour, her postnatal visits are shorter and the patient is left alone more. Like all puerperal women she is apt to worry and possibly to magnify trifles. Her lochia is profuse; or the baby has vomited some food. Should she call the midwife, perhaps in the middle of the night? These and similar problems are easily resolved in hospital, with nursing staff at hand. Serious emergencies such as secondary postpartum haemorrhage, are relatively infrequent, though very worrying if there is delay in getting assistance.

It is clear that the most hazardous time is labour, while the early postnatal period is relatively safe for mother and baby. It follows that to provide the most advantageous conditions for the greatest number of women, there is much to be said in favour of hospital delivery and early transfer home, a practice that continues to gain in popularity.

This question has been answered at some length. Some of the detail could be omitted and a shorter answer would be perfectly adequate.

Questions on this topical subject are being set quite frequently. Examples are given below.

**Q.134. Discuss the factors which should be considered when**

**selecting the place of confinement, and the length of the patient's stay in hospital.**

Here the material is much as that in Q.133, above, but the arrangement differs.

**Q.135. How would you assess the suitability of a patient's home for: (i) home confinement, (ii) early transfer from hospital of a mother and baby?**

This question is altogether different in being of a very practical nature and in concentrating on the social and domestic side of the subject.

**Q.136. Discuss the advantages and disadvantages to mother and baby of early transfer to home from hospital in the postnatal period.**

This question is, in a sense, a distillation of some of the material in Q.133. Its phrasing should be studied with extreme care. The subject is early transfer home; not hospital or home confinement. It would not be difficult to wander from the point.

**Q.137. Discuss the role of the district midwife\* in the care of mothers and babies transferred from hospital within 48 hours of delivery.**

\*The district midwife of 1973, when this question was set, became the community midwife in 1974. This midwife has, in the reorganized health service, become accountable to a different authority. These administrative changes have done little to change the nature of her day-to-day work. It is this practical work, with its various responsibilities, which is the subject of the question.

**Q.138. A multigravid patient is booked for a home confinement.**

**Mention the complications which could arise during labour and the puerperium.**

**What facilities are available in the community to deal with these problems?**

This is a good example of a question which neatly incorporates the medical and social aspects of midwifery. The candidate, in planning her answer, will probably draw upon her experience of multigravid women desiring home confinement, but accepting the hospital booking advised.

**Answer.** No one can forecast categorically that the course of any labour will be absolutely normal. Even in second and third confinements, statistically the safest, complications can arise. In women of higher parity, the risk becomes increasingly greater.

In a rapid labour, the child may be born with no professional attendant present. A multigravid woman, faced with this emergency, is usually quick and sensible, lying down and covering the baby but leaving his face clear. There remains a risk that he may inhale some foreign material or that the airway may be obstructed in some other way.

The mother's uterus may relax and a severe postpartum haemorrhage ensue, with or without a retained placenta.

These hazards can all complicate a precipitate delivery and, additionally, the baby could fall to the floor and receive serious intracranial injury; the cord may snap (though fortunately the damaged vessels do not usually bleed) and the mother may sustain deep perineal lacerations.

Occipito-posterior position may prolong the first stage. In a multigravid woman it is the commonest cause of delay in the second stage, the fetal head being arrested with the occiput lateral, obliquely posterior, or directly posterior. Occasionally a brow or face presentation can develop, probably in the first stage. Cephalopelvic disproportion occurs in some women whose babies are bigger at each confinement.

If the patient has defaulted from clinic, she may now have worsening pre-eclampsia; or a very mobile fetus, with a risk in labour that the cord may prolapse, while a shoulder presentation with a prolapsed arm is not impossible.

Whatever the character of the labour, there is an increased risk of postpartum haemorrhage, a risk which is aggravated if the patient is anaemic.

In women over 35, there is an increased chance of a child having a congenital defect.

The puerperium is somewhat less hazardous, but may still be complicated by uterine subinvolution, with profuse lochia or even a secondary postpartum haemorrhage. Anaemia is common and deep vein thrombosis and even embolus are possibilities.

The community provides numerous facilities for dealing with these problems.

It is quite probable that the patient's family doctor, or the general practitioner obstetrician in the group practice, has been booked, and will be at hand. Failing this, the midwife can call a general practitioner obstetrician under the medical aid scheme.

If either the patient or the baby, or both, must be transferred to hospital, the ambulance service can be called upon. The general practitioner obstetrician is able to call a consultant obstetrician if he finds it necessary, while, if a serious emergency arises, either he or the midwife may call the 'Flying Squad'. This service is available to deal with any emergency arising in the patient's home. The most frequent call is for postpartum haemorrhage, when the 'Flying Squad' will probably resuscitate the patient and, when her condition permits, transfer her to hospital for further treatment. For the mechanical difficulties of labour, it is usual for the patient to be transferred to hospital, rather than to attempt complex operative manoeuvres in the home.

Usually a home help has already been booked. But sometimes the patient's husband is away and she should not be left alone. Or there may be young children in the house, who need care, whether or not the patient goes to hospital. In all these cases the doctor or midwife is able to approach the Social Services Department of the Local Authority, who will make arrangements for the care of the children while the mother is unable to do this herself.

**Q.139. A high parity patient insists on having a home confinement. What arguments would you advance to persuade her to accept**

**hospital confinement?** *(Northern Ireland)*

**Q.140. Why should you persuade a gravida 7, aged 36, who wants to have her baby at home, that she should be delivered in hospital?**

In these two questions the problem is similar to that in Q.134, but here the onus is on the candidate to persuade the patient of the advisability of hospital delivery; and to give the examiner her reasons for doing so. Some candidates might feel happier answering such questions in the first person. This is unimportant; what matters is that cogent and valid arguments shall be adduced.

**Q.141. Write not more than five lines on the importance of each of the following in deciding where a mother should have her third baby:**
    **Her husband's occupation.**
    **Her age.**
    **Her past obstetric history.**
    **Her blood group.**

Over the years the Central Midwives Board has adopted a number of devices to try to elicit short answers. None has been an unqualified success. This is discussed in the section dealing with short answers and this question is included here only on account of its subject matter.

Setting aside the reservation that the five-line requirement shall be met, without benefit of mapping pen, margin or any other 'double parking' ploy, the essential is relevance. In contrast to Q.139 and Q.140, which do rather invite the discursive writer to fill page after page, here every word counts. There is much more time for thinking and planning and every opportunity to reduce the volume of the answer. Here, therefore, an appropriate balance would be twenty minutes planning and ten minutes writing.

**Q.142. What is the value of classes in preparation for childbirth and parentcraft?**

### What subjects should be included in a series of such classes?

Questions about parentcraft appear fairly often in Community Health papers. Sometimes they are straightforward and factual as, e.g., Q.145 below; others have a more nebulous quality which some candidates find off-putting. 'What is the value of . . .' as an opening is a typical example. Of course, any discussion about values has this misty and unmanageable character; it is difficult to know where to start and, once started, it is almost impossible to finish.

The candidate's best plan is to review quickly some of the broader benefits of the classes which she has attended and given; to scribble down three or four *major effects* of the teaching (not *minor details* of the advice given, such as buying well-fitting brassières), to arrange them in reasonable order; pregnancy, labour, puerperium and baby will do well enough if nothing better presents itself; and to write a quite short paragraph about each. This is as much as is reasonable in the time available, which may be calculated to be twenty minutes at the most, since there is a second part to the question.

It is in this second part that the candidate can include some of the material that she was perhaps tempted to classify as 'value'. This is easier, but it is still essential to stick to subjects rather than small details.

**Answer.** The value of classes in preparation for childbirth and parentcraft is much greater than might at first be supposed.

It is obvious that the factual information given – given, as it is, with authority and conviction – will be of value to all expectant mothers. The young primigravida who has learnt some health education and mothercraft at school now acquires a fuller and more personal knowledge. To the older woman who left school twenty years ago, though the subject may be unfamiliar, it is no less interesting. Multigravid women who might have been expected to 'know all the answers' often have misconceptions corrected. Women having a poor obstetric history can often be given genuine hope and encouragement.

Expectant fathers may, on the one hand, have fears and anxieties allayed and, on the other, come to feel an involvement and responsibility. Whether over-protective or too casual, they learn to share the experience and to give their wives support in everything from weighing up the pros and cons of induced labour to washing the dishes.

Independent of all this imparting of information is the value of questions and discussion. In any random group there is one who wants to ask a question, but who hesitates to raise her voice in public. Others have no such inhibition. And when some cheerful extrovert is to be heard asking questions of a highly intimate nature, her more diffident neighbour may well find that her problem, too, is being dealt with. And, such is the nature of group therapy in this situation, that she, too, may gradually come out of her shell.

These groups are, of course, tremendously responsive. This is not surprising when one considers their common interest: every woman in the class looking ahead to what may well be the most momentous occasion in her life. This common bond unites women of widely differing ages and social and ethnic groups in a way that is very salutary in an era of squabbling, fragmentation and dispute.

Finally, it is important to remember that much of the teaching given in parentcraft classes is being disseminated in informal and desultory ways that cannot be assessed accurately. Really interesting classes are discussed long afterwards. Husbands exchange views at work, wives gossip with parents and neighbours and children chatter at school; old wives' tales are shown to be without foundation and superstitions are corrected. Though old ideas die hard, it remains impossible to measure the positive contribution that one series of first-class parentcraft talks can make to the health education of the nation as a whole.

A series of parentcraft classes would deal with the following subjects:

Antenatal clinic: appointments, visits, examinations.

Antenatal advice: diet, exercise, keeping well; minor disorders.

Preparations for baby: clothing, pram, cot, etc.

Arrangements for coming to hospital: clothing, etc., transport, onset of labour.

Preparation for labour: This would vary with the practice of the hospital, classes being given by physiotherapist, obstetrician and midwife. As well as including psychoprophylaxis, relaxation, or any similar procedure, they might cover spontaneous and induced labour, epidural and other analgesics and the role of the husband. Films demonstrating deliveries would be shown and a tour of the hospital would be included.

Care of the baby: washing and bathing; care of the cord and umbilical scar; breast and artificial feeding; minor ailments.

Postnatal care in hospital and at home; self-care procedures; postnatal examination; approach to Family Planning Clinic; Child Welfare Clinic and transfer to care of health visitor.

**Q.143. What is the value of classes in preparation for childbirth and parentcraft?**
**What subjects should be included in a series of such classes?**
*(Northern Ireland)*

This question, set in another country, is identical.

Here is another such question, very similar:

**Q.144. What is the value of classes in preparation for childbirth and parentcraft?**
**What subjects should be included in a series of such classes?**

The same answer would be adequate.

**Q.145. Describe a programme of health education in preparation for parenthood.** *(Scotland)*

Here, as some students might be glad to note, the 'value' factor is omitted and the question concentrates on the programme, which will obviously need to be described in more detail.

Finally, some questions in which a particular aspect of parentcraft is to be considered.

**Q.146. What is the role of the midwife in health education during the antenatal period?**

It will be clear that this question takes in a large proportion of a full parentcraft programme, perhaps the only omission being the informal sessions given in postnatal wards after delivery. Subjects taught by health visitor, obstetrician and physiotherapist should be mentioned for two reasons. Firstly, practice varies so much that, in a particular area, the midwife might be responsible for any or all of these classes. Secondly, the midwife often acts as a co-ordinator in respect of antenatal teaching so her responsibility may come by this route.

Furthermore, the midwife's role is likely to extend beyond a series of classes. Health education in the antenatal period could cover quite an extensive field. It might well include much unplanned material ranging from the patient's questions answered in the antenatal clinic to a discussion in the High Street about the baby's cough.

Even more specialized is Q.147.

**Q.147. Outline a talk to expectant mothers on the immunization facilities available for their babies and give a suggested programme.**

Many candidates, however well they know their basic midwifery, make a list of items to be looked up immediately before the examination. Such a list might include statistics, monetary welfare benefits and possibly immunization programmes. If the candidate is familiar with the subject matter, this answer should present no problems. If not, she can omit this question and answer the other two in Part I of the paper.

**Q.148. In what ways may the midwife help to prepare a primigravida for the emotional and physical aspects of confinement?**

**Q.149. Outline a talk to expectant mothers and fathers on the effect of a first baby on a household.**

These two questions represent two stages in the sequence of material to be covered in parentcraft teaching. The first may be inferred to extend beyond the scope of semi-formal classes alone and certainly needs careful planning. The second is a good deal simpler.

# Short Questions

# Short Questions

Questions of the 'short notes' variety have come to occupy an increasingly prominent place in recent examination papers. The Central Midwives Board for Scotland is very clear in its requirements. The question begins: 'Define the following:' and six terms are to be defined; or, 'What is/are. . . . ?', again requiring a definition or its very near equivalent; or, sometimes, 'Differentiate between . . .', when the candidate is invited to distinguish between pairs of terms which are often confused, e.g., retraction ring and constriction ring. It is incidentally worthy of comment that these 'differentiate' questions are excellent in that they help so much to clarify the candidate's thoughts. The Northern Ireland Council's questions give the candidate a little more latitude. 'Write short notes on *five* of the following . . .', eight subjects being offered, or perhaps short notes on four out of a choice of six subjects. The Central Midwives Board has followed this pattern even more markedly, in that short answers are now expected to occupy one half of the two-hour Community Health paper and no less than two-thirds of the three-hour Midwifery and Paediatrics paper. The examination papers can thus range over a very wide variety of subjects. This has advantages to many candidates, notably the foreign student, who can write down straight facts, but who gets into real difficulties trying to express delicate nuances of meaning; the slow thinker and/or writer, who tends to become embroiled at the construction phase of a longer answer; and the not very knowledgeable candidate, who has forgotten, or never heard of, alpha-fetoprotein or hypernatraemia. It is regrettable to have to omit the answer to a short question; it can be disastrous to fail to answer a longer question.

In the English papers the candidate is usually invited to 'Write about 50 words on each of the following . . .' How is 'about 50 words' to be interpreted? Not less than 45 words or credit will be wasted. In fact, candidates rarely write less than 50 words. But what is the permitted maximum? 55? Most examiners would regard this as very acceptable. 60? Perhaps; but it would be unwise to go beyond this.

In the past, candidates have often disregarded this 'about 50 words' injunction and written answers of 70, 80 or 100 words, occasionally extending to 150 or even 200 words. These regardlessly long answers create so much difficulty in marking that the examiner is hardly to be blamed if he assesses the first fifty or so words with due care and consideration and ignores all the subsequent verbiage. This is stern treatment of the verbose candidate who cannot come to the point; but she should have conformed to her terms of reference.

Moreover, these are not isolated cases. The extent of the problem is to be judged by the measures taken to circumvent it. And so we find, from June 1975, the (one might infer) exasperated addendum seen in questions reproduced on pp. 15 and 17. In fact, the answer must come very close to the 50-word requirement; it is suggested that it should fall within the limits of 45 and 55 words.

Arising from this, the next question the candidate will ask is pertinent enough: 'Is examination time to be occupied/wasted in counting and re-counting words?' Obviously not. The pianist does not check his tempo for the first time at the concert; but he does spend a great deal of time practising. Surely the candidate should prepare herself similarly.

Here are some suggestions.

1. It is necessary to know how many lines of one's own writing amount to 50 words. This, of course, varies, but with small writing it might be 5 or 6 lines and, with a large and sprawling hand perhaps twice as many. Practice will show.

2. Practice may be needed, too, to develop a concise style, squeezing the greatest possible amount of material into the fewest words.

3. Careful tabulation of facts can save words. Sometimes it is appropriate to go further and utilize a chart, as, e.g., in Apgar scoring.

4. At the same time, a balance must be preserved. A grammatical statement can be brief and is often preferable to a page from a notebook, while the use of 'own brand' hospital abbreviations, too

mysterious for the stranger to elucidate, is to be deplored.

5. Diagrams can be extremely valuable in making a point quickly. No examiner will quibble if it is made clear to him at a glance that the candidate has understood what is asked of her and is presenting it as an accurate and correctly labelled picture.

6. Finally, the material. The whole subject – any subject – cannot possibly be covered. Somehow, the candidate must distil the essence of this subject into 50 words. This is, in some respects, the most difficult aspect of the short question. Subjects such as phenylketonuria, ergometrine and neonatal hypothermia might be dealt with fairly adequately in this small compass; but breast feeding, occipitoposterior labour and urinary complications of the puerperium present considerable problems of selection. It may seem paradoxical to state that the better one knows a subject, the easier it becomes to present it concisely; but in some respects, this is certainly true. With greater knowledge comes a sharper sense of proportion. And one important feature of the short answer is not only to know what to put in, but also to know what to leave out.

The candidate who practises consistently on these lines will be very much readier to answer this type of question without wasting time. Indeed, she may well save time since so many of the answers are, as it were, ready made.

The questions that follow, all taken from recent examination papers, have been answered within the condition set: about 50 words. It must be emphasized that this illustrates one way of answering these short questions: not the only way: certainly not the perfect way, if this exists: not necessarily the best way. The student who practises phrasing this type of answer will, in due course, develop the pattern which constitutes the best way for her.

## ANATOMY AND PHYSIOLOGY

### Q.150. The functions of the placenta.

1. Respiratory, oxygen being transmitted from maternal to fetal circulation.
2. Nutritive, nutrients being similarly transmitted.
3. Excretory; carbon dioxide and other waste products pass to

the maternal circulation.
4. Protective: most bacteria cannot pass the placenta. Immune bodies and, less beneficially, viruses can.
5. Endocrine: the placenta, producing oestrogens, progesterone and chorionic gonadotrophin, maintains the pregnancy and prepares for labour.

## Q.151. Moulding of the fetal skull.

Moulding is overlapping of the cranial bones at the sutures and fontanelles enabling the fetal head to adapt to the maternal pelvis.

Slight normal moulding (the sub-occipito-bregmatic and bi-parietal diameters squeezed, the mento-vertical diameter elongated) is harmless; but severe or rapid moulding, especially with compression of the occipito-frontal diameter, can cause intracranial trauma.

## Q.152. Vasa praevia.

Vasa praevia means velamentous vessels from a low-lying placenta crossing the cervix. It is rare but dangerous.

Even with intact membranes the descending head compresses these vessels, causing fetal hypoxia. Ruptured membranes cause ruptured vessels, fetal bleeding and apparent 'antepartum haemorrhage'. Singer's test distinguishes fetal blood and Caesarean section may save the child.

## Q.153. Decidua.

Decidua is endometrium during pregnancy, which, when the blastocyst embeds, becomes thicker and more vascular. The enlarged, closely packed stroma cells form a superficial compact layer; the tortuous, dilated glands create a deeper spongy layer; the basal layer remains unchanged.

Below the blastocyst is basal decidua, around it, capsular decidua and elsewhere, true decidua.

### Q.154. Meconium constituents.

Meconium is a sticky greenish-black material consisting largely of bile and other secretions from the glands in and opening into the alimentary tract. It contains also desquamated epithelial cells from the bowel wall, mucus, and often lanugo hairs, fragments of vernix caseosa and liquor amnii which the fetus has swallowed.


## PREGNANCY

### Q.155. Obesity in pregnancy.

Obesity in pregnancy is undesirable and sometimes hazardous. Accurate blood pressure readings and abdominal and pelvic examinations present difficulty. There is extra strain on the heart and an increased risk of pre-eclampsia. Patients already over-weight cannot be submitted to strict dieting. Patients of normal weight should aim not to gain more than 10 kg during pregnancy.


### Q.156. Engagement of the fetal head.

Engagement of the fetal head means that the maximum pres-enting diameters of the head have passed the plane of the pelvic brim, signifying that brim, cavity and, almost certainly, outlet are adequate. Engagement occurs around the 37th week of a first pregnancy; rather later, possibly after labour begins, in a multi-gravida.


### Q.157. Causes of oedema in pregnancy.

Tissue fluid being normally increased in pregnancy, oedema occurs readily. Slight ankle oedema, settling overnight, is com-mon in well patients. Associated with varicose veins, pre-eclampsia or cardiac disease, it causes increasing concern. More extensive oedema, involving hands, face and occasionally, abdom-inal wall and vulva, occurs in severe pre-eclampsia and eclampsia.

The next three questions recur frequently, with slight variations in wording. Common questions of this kind are well worth memorizing, whether by mnemonic or any other device.

## Q.158. High head at term.

## Q.159. Non-engagement of the fetal head at term.

## Q.160. Causes of non-engagement of the fetal head at term.

Normal factors retarding engagement of the fetal head are multiparity, distension of the bladder or rectum, the supine posture and the high angle of inclination of the pelvic brim in certain ethnic groups.

Abnormal factors are the deflexed head in some occipito-lateral and occipito-posterior positions, placenta praevia, poly-hydramnios and cephalo-pelvic disproportion.

## Q.161. Polyhydramnios.

Polyhydramnios – excessive liquor amnii – is, when marked, recognizable clinically. Typically, about the 32nd week the patient is dyspnoeic, the uterus tense and globular, the fetus mobile and elusive, the heart sounds muffled and a fluid thrill is elicited.

Polyhydramnios, though not fully understood, is associated with monozygotic twin pregnancy, anencephaly, oesophageal atresia and maternal diabetes.

## Q.162. The effects of maternal diabetes on the fetus.

Uncontrolled maternal diabetes can cause abortion, polyhyd-ramnios, excessive fetal growth, fetal oedema and, in late preg-nancy, intra-uterine death. The risk of congenital defect is increased.

In diabetics under specialist care throughout pregnancy the diabetes is very much better stabilized and the likelihood that the fetus will be normal and healthy is strikingly demonstrated.

### Q.163. Transverse lie of the fetus.

This means that the long axis of the fetus lies across the long axis of the uterus. It occurs mainly in women of high parity having poor abdominal and uterine muscle tone. Near term, the treatment is admission, correction to a longitudinal lie and induction of labour to stabilize it. Uncorrected, labour becomes obstructed.

A serious underlying cause, e.g. placenta praevia, must not be overlooked.

### Q.164. Retention of urine at 14 weeks gestation.

This is almost diagnostic of incarceration of the retroverted gravid uterus. The anterior vaginal wall and urethra are elongated and the urethra narrowed. The retention is distressing and increasingly painful.

The patient is hospitalized, an indwelling catheter being introduced. She lies in Sims' position, the foot of the bed raised. The retroversion corrects itself and does not recur.

### Q.165. The dangers of essential hypertension in pregnancy.

A mildly hypertensive patient may go through pregnancy without adverse effect, either to herself or the fetus. The fetus may be small.

In moderate, worsening and severe hypertension the mother is at risk of pre-eclampsia, sub-arachnoid haemorrhage and abruptio placentae, with their complications.

With placental insufficiency, the hazards to the fetus are smallness for dates and intra-uterine death.

**Q.166. Ultrasonic examination.**

By ultrasound scan single or multiple pregnancy is revealed by the 10th week; placental localization before amniocentesis, or to detect placenta praevia, is possible; congenital central nervous system defects are recognized; with Sonicaid apparatus fetal movements are seen, fetal heart sounds are heard by the 10th week and deep vein thrombosis is recognizable.

**Q.167. Painless vaginal bleeding at 33 weeks gestation.**

This painless bleeding may be from placenta praevia, placental abruption, or cervical or vaginal lesions.

The patient is hospitalized. Speculum examination reveals local lesions. If available, ultrasound scan shows the situation of the placenta.

Often the bleeding is slight and transient. Should it increase, blood transfusion and Caesarean section might become necessary.

**Q.168. Vaginal discharge in pregnancy.**

Slight non-irritating vaginal discharge (from increased activity of the cervical glands) is normal. Thick cheesy discharge with intense irritation indicates monilial vaginitis. Frothy irritating discharge occurs in trichomonad vaginitis. Gonorrhoea, sometimes symptomless, can cause thin greenish discharge, skin excoriation and severe urethritis with scalding. Blood staining occurs in carneous mole and severe vaginitis.

**Q.169. Bleeding per vaginam in the first 12 weeks of pregnancy.**

Bleeding per vaginam before the 12th week may be nidation bleeding, bleeding from the decidual space, extra-uterine bleeding or associated with ectopic pregnancy, but most commonly it is due to abortion.

In threatened abortion the bleeding is slight and painless. If it is severe, especially with pain from uterine contractions, abortion is inevitable.

### Q.170. Amniocentesis.

In amniocentesis, the amniotic sac is punctured via the abdomen, to give a fetal intraperitoneal transfusion or to withdraw amniotic fluid for one of the following tests:
(a) chromosome investigation for trisomies.
(b) lecithin/sphingomyelin ratio for lung development.
(c) bilirubin concentration (serially) in Rhesus iso-immunization.
(d) alpha-feto-protein concentration in suspect central nervous system defect.

### Q.171. Asymptomatic bacteriuria.

Asymptomatic bacteriuria is potentially serious. All pregnant women should be screened; about 10 per cent will be positive.
It is diagnosed when a count reveals 100,000 or more bacteria in 1 ml of urine.
Of affected patients, 25 per cent are anticipated to develop symptoms, sometimes severe and occasionally leading to death.
All affected patients should therefore be treated.

## LABOUR

### Q.172. Principles of the delivery of the second twin.

These principles are:
1. Diagnosis in time to withhold the routine oxytocic drug.
2. At the earliest moment, checking the lie: correcting to longitudinal if necessary.
3. Rupturing the membranes to limit delay as the placental oxygen supply soon diminishes. After 15 minutes assisted delivery

is recommended.
4. Avoiding precipitate delivery with its risk of intracranial trauma.

### Q.173. The tissues cut when an episiotomy is performed.

The tissues cut in medio-lateral episiotomy are perineal skin, fibres of bulbocavernosus, superficial and deep transverse perineal muscles, probably fibres of the pubo-vaginalis portion of pubo-coccygeus and vaginal epithelium.

If subsequent repair is to safeguard the integrity of the pelvic floor, the muscles, layer by layer, must be brought into apposition and efficiently sutured.

### Q.174. Causes of delay in the second stage of labour.

### Q.175. Causes of delay in the second stage.

Another recurring question.
1. Insufficiently strong contractions and/or failure of a deflexed head fully to rotate, the occiput being lateral, obliquely posterior or persistently posterior.
2. Face or breech presentation.
3. Slight outlet disproportion or an unyielding perineum delays the perineal phase.
4. Failure to 'push' causes slight delay.
5. Rare causes are a short cord or a constriction ring.

### Q.176. The importance of examination of the placenta and membranes.

### Q.177. Why must you examine the placenta and membranes following delivery?

The placenta and membranes are examined, primarily to determine their completeness. Retained placental tissue causes bleeding, often severe. Retained chorion favours bacterial growth, thus contributing to puerperal infection.

Types of twins may be determined by exact examination of placenta and membranes.

A cord having only two vessels arouses suspicion of renal abnormality in the child.

In these specimen answers, the questions have been written above, since the student has no question paper to refer to. In the examination the candidate is asked not to write out the question.

Questions 176 and 177 are good examples of the time wasted by a candidate having a 'blind spot' who insists on copying the questions. One or two words at the beginning of a short question are immaterial. One or two lines may constitute a quarter of the 50 words requested and should thus be omitted at all costs.

### Q.178. Mendelsohn's syndrome.

Mendelsohn's syndrome occurs when, during anaesthesia, regurgitated gastric contents are inhaled. The acidity irritates the pulmonary epithelium, causing bronchospasm, pulmonary oedema and respiratory failure.

Prophylaxis. During labour food and dextrose drinks are withheld. Mist. magnesium trisilicate is given 3 to 4 hourly. During anaesthesia, cuffed endotracheal tubes and cricoid pressure are employed to prevent inhalation of irritants.

### Q.179. Primary postpartum haemorrhage.

This is excessive bleeding from the genital tract within 24 hours of delivery. 'Excessive' means 300 ml or more: less if it adversely affects the mother's condition. The commonest cause is inadequate uterine contraction during or after the third stage. The immediate treatment is 'rubbing up' a contraction and administering 0·5 mg intravenous ergometrine. Traumatic postpartum haemorrhage is uncommon.

**Q.180. Fetal scalp blood sampling.**

Fetal scalp blood sampling permits accurate assessment of suspect and impending fetal hypoxia.

Via an endoscope the fetal scalp is cleansed, minutely incised, capillary blood withdrawn into a heparinized tube and its pH value determined by Astrup micro-apparatus. Normally above $7 \cdot 25$, values between $7 \cdot 25$ and $7 \cdot 20$ indicate increasing hypoxia and below $7 \cdot 20$ the need for immediate delivery.


Another recurring question:

**Q.181. The recognition of fetal distress in labour.**

**Q.182. Fetal distress in labour.**

Fetal distress (fetal hypoxia) in labour is shown clinically by fetal heart rate variations: transient tachycardia, 140–156, increasing bradycardia, 156–140–132, and irregularity. Meconium stained liquor is suspicious. The fetal scalp blood pH gives precise information: at pH $7 \cdot 25$ delivery is necessary, at pH $7 \cdot 20$ urgently so, and forceps delivery or Caesarean section is undertaken.


**Q.183. Indications for vaginal examination during labour.**

Indications for vaginal examination:
1. To determine normal progress:
(a) To ascertain if labour has begun;
(b) Identity, position and station of presenting part;
(c) State of membranes and liquor;
(d) Serially, to measure progress;
2. To ascertain the cause of delay in first or second stage.
3. To decide if a retained placenta is in the vagina.

**Q.184. Deep transverse arrest of the fetal head.**

In this common cause of second stage delay, the deflexed head is arrested deep in the pelvis, the occipito-frontal diameter transversely between the ischial spines. Often this interspinous diameter is narrowed and the uterine contractions insufficiently strong. The treatment, Kielland's forceps rotation and extraction, is carried out under pudendal nerve block.

**Q.185. The presence of the husband in the labour ward.**

If both desire it, the duly prepared husband should be present. He is a comforting, reassuring first stage companion, often interested in the monitoring apparatus. During delivery he should sit down, holding his wife's hand. A photographic enthusiast may film the delivery. For forceps delivery, or in any other abnormality, he should probably withdraw.

**Q.186. The significance during labour of a narrow sub-pubic arch.**

This signifies two possibilities:
1. Severe perineal lacerations. In the second stage the fetal head, sometimes occipito-posterior, is forced backwards. Early and adequate episiotomy is needed.
2. Outlet disproportion. Unless progress is good, a trial of forceps (in a theatre prepared for Caesarean section) enables the obstetrician to decide whether vaginal delivery is feasible or Caesarean section preferable.


**THE PUERPERIUM**

**Q.187. The reasons for early ambulation in puerperium.**

Early ambulation is beneficial in improving pelvic and leg circulation, helping to avoid venous thrombosis. Bed-pans are abolished, facilitating micturition and defaecation. The mother probably prefers perineal self-care and enjoys a bath or shower and attending to her baby. Being 'up and about' engenders well-being and eases the subsequent return to housewife status.

## Q.188. Pulmonary embolism in the puerperium.

Puerperal pulmonary embolism is dangerous and occasionally fatal. The cause may be unknown. It can follow Caesarean section, thrombophlebitis or, occasionally, oestrogen therapy.

Three to four days after delivery the patient has severe constricting chest pain, dyspnoea, hypotension, possibly haemoptysis and cardiac arrest.

Treatment may include external cardiac massage, oxygen, anticoagulants and often antibiotics.

## Q.189. Superficial thrombophlebitis.

Superficial thrombophlebitis is predisposed to by increased blood viscosity, varicosities, dehydration and haemorrhage in labour, age (over 35), high parity and lack of activity.

With low-grade pyrexia, the affected vein is tender and painful, the skin reddened.

Treatment: elevation of the leg and exercises; walking, wearing support tights.

Pulmonary embolus is unlikely.

## Q.190. Puerperal depression.

Many women experience a transitory unhappy, tearful phase three to four days after delivery, recovering quickly. A few, sleepless and despondent, become withdrawn, developing puerperal depression and needing psychiatric treatment.

Prophylaxis. Emotional instability is anticipated, 'tender loving care' and sympathetic listening are needed and insomnia is sought and remedied.

When necessary, a psychiatrist is consulted promptly.

## Q.191. Engorged breasts.

Breast engorgement, common on the third or fourth postnatal day, is uncomfortable and sometimes painful, with slight pyrexia. The breasts should be emptied, by the baby or by gentle hand or machine expressing. A binder may be applied and fluids restricted. Oestrogens are avoided.

Unilateral engorgement with a flushed breast and pyrexia denotes mastitis.

## Q.192. What complications involving the urinary tract can arise in the puerperium?

Puerperal complications involving the urinary tract are:
1. Urinary retention: complete, residual, or with overflow.
2. Urinary incontinence, either retention with overflow, as above, or, rarely, from a vesico-vaginal fistula.
3. Urinary tract infection may complicate urinary retention or a pre-existing infection may recur.
4. Rarely, renal failure may complicate abruptio placentae, hypofibrinogenaemia, or eclampsia.

## Q.193. Causes of pyrexia in the puerperium.

Apart from transient 'reactionary' pyrexia following long or difficult labour, the two commonest causes of pyrexia in the puerperium are:
1. Urinary tract infection.
2. Genital tract infection.
   Other causes are:
3. Severe breast engorgement.
4. Mastitis.
5. Thrombophlebitis.

The possibility of an intercurrent infection such as influenza must not be overlooked.

## Q.194. Abnormal lochia.

Excessive, persistently red lochia occurs with retained placental tissue. It may assume the proportions of secondary postpartum haemorrhage.

Excessive reddish-brown lochia is noted when the uterus is subinvoluted.

Profuse brown lochia, sometimes offensive, occurs with retained membrane and local uterine infection.

Scanty or suppressed lochia with high pyrexia signifies puerperal septicaemia.

## Q.195. Postnatal insomnia.

Much contributes to postnatal insomnia: excitement, unfamiliar surroundings, noise, pain, anxiety. It is usually remedied by good nursing and sedative or analgesic drugs.

Insomnia is never ignored since it is the first evidence of impending mental disorder. Any patient sleeping badly, especially if she herself is uncomplaining, should without delay be seen by a psychiatrist.

## Q.196. Postnatal exercises.

Postnatal exercises, particularly in the first few days after delivery, help to restore pelvic floor and abdominal muscle tone. They improve the pelvic and leg circulation, lessening the likelihood of venous thrombosis. By improving posture, exercises decrease sacro-iliac strain and the backache which it causes. They create a sense of well-being and hasten rehabilitation.

## Q.197. What is the value of a postnatal examination at the sixth week?

The sixth week postnatal examination is valuable in that:
(a) sub-involution and cervicitis are diagnosed and may be

treated. Cervical cytology can be undertaken.
(b)  pelvic floor integrity can be checked.
(c)  anaemias may be detected and treated.
(d)  advice can be given on rest, return to work, baby care and feeding and family planning.

### Q.198. Care of the perineum.

First the midwife performs the perineal toilet, then the patient learns self-care. She baths or uses a bidet with hand-spray and learns to dry the perineum and apply a sterile pad without risking contamination. The midwife daily inspects lochia and perineum and removes non-absorbable sutures on the 6th postnatal day.

## THE NEW-BORN CHILD

### Q.199. Identification of the newborn.

Before the child's removal from the delivery bed, the mother's identity is checked, identical wristlets being put on her and the baby and the cot labelled. Hand and/or footprints are sometimes taken.

These identifications remain throughout the stay in hospital, being checked whenever the child is moved to or from the cot.

### Q.200. The Guthrie test.

The Guthrie test, routine on the 6th neonatal day, excludes (once in 10,000 cases detects) phenylketonuria. This inborn error of metabolism causes mental retardation unless a specific diet is given.

The midwife, by heel prick, collects four drops of blood on treated absorbent paper. The test, dependent on the growth of bacteria, is deferred if the child is receiving antibiotics.

**Q.201. Neonatal hypoxia.**

Neonatal hypoxia occurs when initiation of respiration is delayed and/or if respiratory distress syndrome develops. It may follow intra-uterine hypoxia. This prolonged hypoxic interval can lead to physical or mental handicap.

Endotracheal intubation, intermittent positive pressure respiration and correction of blood chemistry are necessary.

**Q.202. Care of a preterm baby during transfer to a specialized unit.**

An experienced midwife accompanies the preterm child during transfer.

A clear airway is maintained, oxygen and suction apparatus being at hand.

To avoid chilling, a heated incubator and non-conductive wrappers are needed.

Equipment is sterile and the route taken during transfer is preferably uncontaminated.

The child, separated from the mother, is readily identifiable.

**Q.203. Anti-D gamma globulin.**

In Rhesus iso-immunization the fetal cells which stimulate maternal antibody production enter the mother's circulation as the placenta separates. An injection of anti-D gamma globulin given shortly after labour destroys fetal cells before the D-antigen they contain invokes antibody production.

The effect being transient, the gamma globulin is given to all Rh-negative mothers after every delivery or abortion.

**Q.204. Oral thrush in the newborn.**

In this common condition, neonatal moniliasis, adherent white patches occur inside the mouth and on the tongue. The child, whether breast or artificially fed, is hungry but reluctant to feed and sucking appears painful. Often the mother has had vaginal moniliasis in pregnancy. The treatment is oral Nystatin, 1–500, 5 ml b.d. The mother's hand-washing practice may be at fault.

### Q.205. Oesophageal atresia.

Oesophageal atresia, often with accompanying tracheo-oesphageal fistula, is a congenital defect. The fetus cannot swallow, polyhydramnios results and though at birth the child appears normal or perhaps excessively 'mucus-y', oesophageal patency must be determined. The affected neonate is not fed orally and is quickly transferred to a children's hospital for surgery.

### Q.206. The advantages of breast feeding.

Breast feeding, being normal, natural, physiological and usually easy, should not need advocating. However, advantages can be adduced:

It supplies all nutritional needs exactly; and the emotional needs of mothering, cuddling and security.

Specific antibodies protect the child from E. coli and other infections.

Breast-fed babies are less liable to respiratory infections, cot deaths, obesity and metabolic disorders.

### Q.207. Diarrhoea among babies in a maternity ward.

More than one case of diarrhoea among neonates suggests gastroenteritis and necessitates immediate action.

Affected babies are rigidly isolated and treated. The ward is closed to admissions. The source of the infection is sought among mothers and medical, nursing and ancillary staff. The ward is emptied and disinfected before admissions are resumed.

## Q.208. What do you understand by Apgar scoring of the newborn?

Virginia Apgar, an American paediatrician, recommended assessment one and five minutes after birth, on five vital signs, as follows:

**Apgar score showing typical normal rating**

| Score | 0 | 1 | 2 | Minutes 1 | 5 |
|---|---|---|---|---|---|
| Heart beat | Absent | Less than 100 | 100 + | 2 | 2 |
| Respiratory effort | Nil | Weak/ irregular | Strong cry | 1 | 2 |
| Colour | Greyish white | Trunks pink Limbs blue | Completely pink | 1 | 2 |
| Muscle tone | Limp | Some flexion of limbs | Active | 2 | 2 |
| Response to stimulus | Nil | Poor | Brisk | 2 | 2 |
| | | | Totals | 8 | 10 |

e.g. 0–4 = condition poor; 5–7 = condition fair; 8–10 = condition good.

An Apgar score, correctly set out together with an example of its use, illustrates this answer in relatively few words. The student might well write a description without the chart, in order to decide which method is the more concise.

## Q.209. Care of the stump of the umbilical cord.

In one common procedure a Hollister clamp is applied, flush with the umbilicus, and the stump shortened and swabbed with 1 per cent chlorhexidine in spirit. The swabbing is repeated and Sterzac powder applied twice daily until separation and healing have occurred.

If routine twice daily inspection reveals redness or 'stickiness', 4-hourly swabbings are started.

## Q.210. Hypocalcaemia in the newborn.

Hypocalcaemia, a fall to 7·5 mg/100 ml or less in serum calcium occurs in some babies given cows' milk mixtures. The high phosphate content can delay calcium absorption and, at 6 to 8 days, the child becomes irritable, with muscular twitchings and, occasionally, convulsions.

The condition is quickly reversed by giving calcium gluconate or calcium syrup.

## Q.211. Ophthalmia neonatorum.

Ophthalmia neonatorum is any purulent conjunctivitis occurring within 21 days of birth. Formerly notifiable, it occurs commonly as a transient 'sticky eye' a few days after birth. A swab is taken and antibiotic ointment or drops may be started. Occasionally severe staphylococcal or gonococcal ophthalmia occurs with risk of corneal ulceration and impaired vision.

## COMMUNITY HEALTH

### Q.212. Perinatal mortality.

Perinatal deaths are stillbirths and deaths in the first week of life. The perinatal mortality rate is the number of such deaths per thousand registered live and stillbirths in any one year: in 1975, 19·2.

The principal causes are low birth weight, hypoxia, asphyxia neonatorum, intracranial birth trauma and severe congenital defects.

### Q.213. Genetic counselling.

Genetic counselling is expert information and advice available to couples who have or might anticipate having children with chromosomal abnormalities such as Down's syndrome and certain inborn errors of metabolism. If the parents are aware of a known high risk they can discuss the matter and be helped in their decision whether or not to have further children.

### Q.214. Emergency obstetric unit ('Obstetric Flying Squad')

This 'Flying Squad' is a fully equipped, experienced team – obstetrician, anaesthetist and midwife – available to doctors and midwives for domiciliary obstetric emergencies.

Calls are principally for haemorrhages: sometimes for eclampsia or mechanical problems.

The patient is first resuscitated, then transferred to hospital for treatment. Blood transfusion is preferably deferred until full cross-matching is completed.

### Q.215. Immunization programme for children up to five years of age.

Recommended programme, slight variation being acceptable.

Three doses of triple vaccine (diphtheria/tetanus/pertussis) and oral poliomyelitis vaccine at age six, eight and twelve months.

One dose of measles vaccine at thirteen months.

A 'booster' dose of poliomyelitis vaccine at school entrance.

Smallpox vaccination is no longer recommended. World-wide eradication is envisaged shortly.

### Q.216. Family planning services.

Family planning services, provided by Area Health Authorities, are clinics where advice, examination and contraceptive materials are offered free to married and unmarried women, on medical and social grounds. Patients are informed shortly after delivery or earlier. The 6th week postnatal examination may be combined with a family planning clinic visit.


## Q.217. District Management Team.

The District Management Team comprises the District Community Physician, District Nursing Officer, District Finance Officer, District Administrator, a local consultant and a general practitioner and supporting professional staff.

This team co-ordinates work delegated by the Area Health Authority to the District, namely the management of hospital and community services at patient level.

## Q.218. Area Health Authorities.

Area Health Authorities are operational authorities in the Health Service, accountable to Regional Health Authorities and responsible for assessing Area needs and planning, administering and delegating to Districts appropriate health care.

England has 90 such authorities, having their boundaries co-terminous with those of non-metropolitan counties, metropolitan districts and groups of 2 to 3 London Boroughs.


## Q.219. Community Health Councils.

Community Health Councils are lay committees of 20 to 25 members, set up by Area Health Authorities, one to each District and responsible for representing the interests of patients in that District. They thus express consumer opinion about, e.g., patient care, transport or other facilities, and make appropriate recommendations to the Area Health Authority.


## MISCELLANEOUS

### Q.220. Define the following:
(a) **Haemolytic disease of the newborn**
(b) **Haemorrhagic disease of the newborn**

(c) **Transverse lie**
(d) **Deep transverse arrest**
(e) **Involution of the uterus**
(f) **Inversion of the uterus.**

If the candidate knows her subject well and is familiar with the appropriate definitions, this answer can be completed in a very few minutes.

Two important facts should be noted: firstly, that all definitions, as the term itself indicates, should be exact and definite: and, it might be added, as brief as is consistent with clarity. Secondly, and in this question particularly, precise definitions clear up confusion between incorrectly used and misunderstood terms. The terms set out above are presented in pairs: pairs that do indeed create confusion in many minds. Thus, like many other examination questions, this one has a twofold aim, not only to test the candidate's knowledge, but to help to clarify it.

**Answer.** (a) Haemolytic disease of the newborn is most often seen as a condition resulting from blood incompatibility, between parents of different ABO groups or Rhesus types, in which the child's blood undergoes marked haemolysis resulting in anaemia, jaundice and, in severe cases, brain damage.

(b) Haemorrhagic disease of the newborn is a condition of unknown aetiology, in which the infant, born with a very low blood prothrombin value, suffers apparently spontaneous haemorrhages from mucus membranes, causing, most often, haematemesis and melaena neonatorum.

(c) Transverse lie means that the longitudinal axis of the fetus lies transversely across the longitudinal axis of the mother's uterus.

(d) Deep transverse arrest means that the fetus lies longitudinally with the vertex presenting, the sagittal suture positioned transversely across the pelvic outlet at the level of the ischial spines. Progress is arrested because the head is deflexed, the spines prominent and probably the uterine contractions insufficiently strong.

(e) By involution of the uterus is meant the return of this organ following labour to its pre-pregnant state. The process of autolysis whereby this is brought about takes eight or ten weeks.

(f) Inversion of the uterus means a turning of the uterus inside out; it occurs generally in the mismanaged third stage, when, the placenta not being fully separated and the uterus not contracting, cord traction is exerted or fundal pressure is applied; it is very traumatic and produces deep shock.

**Q.221. Differentiate between:**
**(a) Perimetrium and Parametrium**
**(b) Retraction Ring and Constriction Ring**
**(c) Presentation and Presenting Part**
**(d) Inevitable and Incomplete Abortion**
**(e) Quickening and Lightening.** *(Scotland)*

It is understandable that these perhaps quaintly named terms should sometimes create confusion, particularly in the mind of the student whose mother tongue is not English.

In answering questions of this kind, definitions are certainly needed, but the answer must go beyond this, to show the essential difference between each term and its counterpart.

(a) *Perimetrium* is the peritoneal covering of the uterus.

*Parametrium* is the pelvic cellular tissue lying adjacent to the uterus: mainly lateral to the body and cervix of the uterus, below and between the folds of the broad ligaments.

(b) The *Retraction Ring* is a ridge running round the uterus. It marks the difference in thickness between the thick strongly retracted upper uterine segment in advanced labour and the thin, stretched lower segment. Only if labour is obstructed, with extreme retraction, does the retraction ring rise out of the pelvis, to become palpable abdominally. The term Bandl's Ring is probably synonymous, though some authorities restrict its use to obstructed labour.

A *Constriction Ring* is a narrow, tight ring at one level in the uterus. It is a ring of tonically contracted muscle, possibly gripping the fetus round the neck, or, in the third stage (when the self-explanatory expression 'hourglass' constriction is used) preventing expulsion of the placenta.

(c) The *Presentation* is the part of the fetus which enters the pelvis first: usually the vertex, but sometimes the breech or face.

The *Presenting Part* is that part of the fetus lying immediately over the internal os, and the first part to be palpated during vaginal examination. Normally it is the posterior part of the parietal bone which lies anteriorly in the pelvis and over which the caput forms.

(d) *Inevitable Abortion* is abortion which has progressed to a stage when it cannot be arrested. The uterine contractions have caused the cervix to begin dilating.

*Incomplete Abortion* (a sub-division of inevitable abortion) is a stage at which part, but not all, of the products of conception has been expelled from the uterus. Usually the fetus is expelled and the placenta retained, with serious risks of haemorrhage and infection.

(e) *Quickening* describes the time when a patient first feels fetal movements: in a first pregnancy, 18–20 weeks; in subsequent pregnancies, about 16 weeks.

*Lightening* occurs about the 36–37th week, when the presenting part of the fetus begins to descend into the pelvis and the fundus is lower in the abdomen. The lungs and upper abdomen are less compressed, breathing is easier and the patient experiences a sense of relief.

In these two last questions, simple diagrams might save time. Transverse lie and transverse arrest, retraction and constriction ring and inevitable and incomplete abortion can all be illustrated quickly by a candidate who may have little artistic talent but who has a good photographic memory.